Urology

A Handbook for Medical Students

Urology

A Handbook for Medical Students

S. Brewster, D. Cranston, J. Noble and J. Reynard

Consultant Urologists, Department of Urology, The Churchill Hospital, Oxford, UK

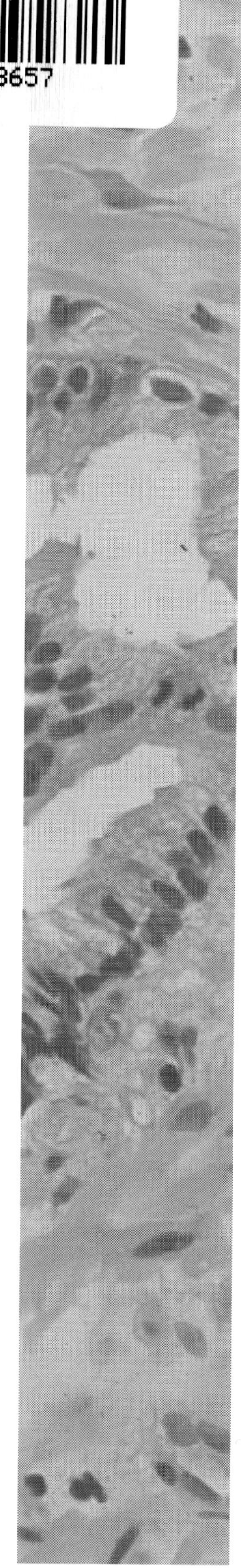

BIOS

First published 2001

A CIP catalogue record for this book is available from the British Library.

ISBN 1 85996 300 5

BIOS Scientific Publishers Ltd
9 Newtec Place, Magdalen Road, Oxford OX4 1RE, UK
Tel. +44 (0)1865 726286. Fax +44 (0)1865 246823
World Wide Web home page: http://www.bios.co.uk/

Production Editor: Sarah Carlson
Typeset by Creative Associates, Oxford, UK
Printed by TJ International Ltd, Padstow, UK

Contents

Abbreviations

AAA – abdominal aortic aneurysm
AAT – androgen ablation therapy
ACE – angiotensin-converting enzyme
AFP – alpha-fetoprotein
AML – angiomyolipoma
ATG – anti-thymocyte globulin
ATN – acute tubular necrosis
AUA – American Urological Association
BCG – bacilli Calmette–Guerin
BCR – bulbocavernosus reflex
BNI – bladder neck incision
BOO – bladder outflow (outlet) obstruction
BPE – benign prostatic enlargement
BPH – benign prostatic hyperplasia
BPO – benign prostatic obstruction
BXO – balanitis xerotica obliterans
CAH – congenital adrenal hyperplasia
CAPD – chronic ambulatory peritoneal dialysis
CIS – carcinoma in-situ
CMV – cytomegalovirus
CRF – chronic renal failure
CT – computerized tomography
CTU – CT urography
CVA – cerebrovascular accident
DESD – detrusor-external sphincter dyssynergia
DGD – D-glycerate dehydrogenase
DHT – dihydrotestosterone
DMSA – dimercapto-succinic acid
DRE – digital rectal examination
EBRT – external beam radiotherapy
ED – erectile dysfunction
EMU – early morning urine
ESR – erythrocyte sedimentation rate
ESRF – end stage renal failure
ESWL – extracorporeal shock wave lithotripsy
FSH – follicle stimulating hormone
GU – genito-urinary
hCG – human chorionic gonadotrophin
HIV – human immunodeficiency virus
HLA – human leucocyte antigen
HPV – human papilloma virus
ICSI – intracytoplasmic sperm injection
IPSS – International Prostate Symptom Score
ISC – intermittent self catheterization
IVC – inferior vena cava
IVF – in-vitro fertilization
IVU – intravenous urogram
KUB – kidneys, ureter and bladder
LDH – lactate dehydrogenase

LH – leuteinizing hormone
LRD – living related donor
LURD – living unrelated donor
LUTS – lower urinary tract symptoms
MAG3 – mercaptoacetyl-triglycyl
MCUG – micturating cystourethrogram
MESA – microsurgical epididymal sperm aspiration
MHC – major histocompatibility complex
MRI – magnetic resonance imaging
MSK – medullary sponge kidney
MSU – mid-stream urine
PC – prostate cancer
PCNL – percutaneous nephrolithotomy
PGE1 – prostoglandin E1
PIN – prostatic intraepithelial neoplasia
PPV – patent processus vaginalis
PSA – prostate specific antigen
PUJ – pelvi-ureteric junction
PUV – posterior urethral valves
PZ – peripheral zones
Q_{max} – maximal flow rate
RCC – renal cell carcinoma
SARS – sacral anterior root stimulator
SUZI – subzonal sperm injection
TC – testicular cancer
TCC – transitional cell carcinoma
TESA – testicular sperm aspiration
TOV – trial of void
TRUS – transrectal ultrasonography
TS – tuberous sclerosis
TSE – testicular self-examination
TUR – transurethral resection
TURP – transurethral resection of the prostate
TUU – transureteroureterostomy
TWOC – trial without catheter
UDT – undescended testis
USS – ultrasound scan
UTI – urinary tract infection
VCMG – videocystometrography
VHL – von Hippel Lindau
VUR – vesico-ureteric reflux

Preface

Urology as a surgical speciality has been evolving for over 200 years. In most UK hospitals, it was practised by general surgeons until the 1970s, when new and replacement appointments for dedicated urological surgeons became normal procedure. Higher surgical training in urology is now entirely separate from general surgery. After basic surgical training has been completed, 5 years is spent as Specialist Registrar with the attainment of the specialist FRCS (urol.) examination. Urology continues to evolve, keeping pace with technological advances such as fibre optic endoscopy, laser and laparoscopic instrumentation, therapeutics and molecular biology.

Often describing themselves to patients as 'human plumbers', urologists diagnose and treat surgical conditions of the male genito-urinary tract and the female urinary tract. Hence tumours, stones, infections and obstruction form the majority of his or her workload. However, the urologist becomes involved with endocrinology, medical oncology, nephrology, neurology and fertility medicine on occasions. While few of the conditions are life threatening, urological problems account for about 25% of emergency surgical admissions to hospital, acute retention of urine and ureteric colic being the common ones. Fifteen percent of doctors will suffer from a stone in the urinary tract at some stage in their life.

The British Association of Urological Surgeons (BAUS) is the professional organization of the speciality. BAUS recommends one consultant per 100 000 people. Most European countries have a ratio of 1:50 000 or less. The USA has a ratio of 1:29 000. At present, we fall short of target, at 1:130 000 in the UK, so there is a need for expansion.

This is currently the only book expressly written for medical students entirely by practising urologists. We hope that through the text and illustrations, the recommendations for further reading, the case studies and the key points boxes featured in each of the 12 chapters, we have covered emergency and elective urology and given a taster for some of the recent advances and current controversies. Of course, no book can replace the practical experience of history taking and examination skills that must be learnt in the clinic or on the ward; neither does this book deal in depth with surgical detail that would be more relevant to a surgical trainee. We hope that you enjoy the book and your clinical attachment in urology. If you wish to suggest potential improvements of a future edition, please write to or e-mail us simon.brewster@orh.anglox.nhs.uk) – we will be grateful for your feedback.

Finally, we wish to thank Mr Griff Fellows for providing some of the illustrations and Dr Rebecca Pollard for reviewing the draft manuscript.

CHAPTER 1

Urological history and examination

Taking a urological history

Patients with urological complaints can be of any age, physical and mental disposition, either (or both) sex, and hail from every social background imaginable. Take an incomplete history, ignoring the social side and you will miss men and women who have fought at sea in the Battle of Jutland, on land in the mud of Ypres, flew on the Dambusters raid, served corgis aboard the Royal Yacht and acted as the Queen's chauffeur. The consultation should, as always, start with introductions and the offer of a handshake, after which its own flavour will develop. Like other surgical long cases, the consultation should take about 20 minutes. The complaint may be of an emergency nature, in which case analgesia or other pain-relieving treatment should be available as soon as the cause of the problem is established. If the patient wishes, any interested accompanying relative or supporter should be encouraged to be present during the history-taking and final discussion.

The patient's **age** and **occupation** (or former occupation if retired) are noted. The occupation is important because it may give a clue to the diagnosis: for example, someone complaining of haematuria working for 20 years in a tyre factory probably has bladder cancer.

The **presenting complaint** is noted, its duration, associated symptoms and the impact it is having on the patient's life. The commonest complaints in urology are lower urinary tract symptoms and haematuria.

Lower urinary tract symptoms (LUTS) can be divided into two groups, as shown in *Table 1.1*. When considering LUTS, it is relevant to note whether storage or voiding symptoms predominate. Finally, an assessment of the 'bother' or disruption to daily activity or sleep as a result of the LUTS is worthwhile: this helps later when discussing treatment options. Symptom scores are described on page 36.

Haematuria may be painless or associated with loin, abdominal or urethral pain. Total haematuria

Table 1.1:
Lower urinary tract symptoms and haematuria

Storage (filling)	Voiding (obstructive)	Haematuria
Daytime frequency (try to ascertain the number)	Hesitancy (waiting to start void)	Painless
Nocturia (an average number is helpful)	Reduced flow pressure (compared to the past)	Painful (loin or urethral)
Urgency ± incontinence	Post-micturition dribble	Total (throughout voiding)
Strangury (urethral pain at the end of voiding)	Intermittent flow (stopping and starting)	Initial (only at the start of voiding)
Suprapubic pain	Feeling of incomplete emptying	Terminal (only at the end of voiding)
	Pneumaturia (passage of gas)	
	Faecaluria (passage of faecal debris)	
	Dysuria (urethral pain during voiding)	

Table 1.2:
The causes of haematuria

General medical causes	Kidney	Ureter	Bladder	Urethra incl. prostate
Coagulation disorders	Tumour	Tumour	Tumour	Tumour
Beetroot	Stone	Stone	Stone	Stone
Exercise	Trauma	Trauma	Trauma	Trauma
Drugs e.g. warfarin	Infection		Infection	Infection
Drugs e.g. warfarin glomerulonephritis	Arteriovenous malformation, renal artery aneurysm		Foreign body	Foreign body
			Idiopathic, bladder neck	Idiopathic, prostate
	Papillary necrosis			

implies bleeding from the kidneys, ureters or bladder. Initial haematuria is likely to be prostatic or urethral and terminal haematuria is more likely to be from the bladder neck. Haematuria with pain implies stone or infection; painless haematuria implies either tumour or benign renal or prostatic bleeding. The causes of haematuria are shown in *Table 1.2*.

Haematospermia is an uncommon complaint. Usually painless, careful questioning is required to ensure the reported blood has not come from the sexual partner or the patients' urine. Associated pain implies the presence of a prostatic inflammation or calculus. It tends to be self-limiting, but requires investigation (urine stick-test, cysto-urethroscopy, serum prostate specific antigen [PSA] if persistent.

Incontinence is the involuntary urethral loss of urine. Incontinence is covered in Chapter 5, but for the purpose of history-taking, it may be divided into:

(a) nocturnal enuresis (bedwetting);
(b) stress incontinence, only associated with physical activity such as sneezing;
(c) urge incontinence, associated with urgency (the urgent desire to pass urine);
(d) total incontinence, associated with overflow of a desensitized bladder or from a non-functioning urinary sphincter mechanism.

The complaint of **pain** should trigger a set of questions regarding its nature: site, severity, duration, constancy, radiation, aggravating factors, relieving factors, whether there has been previous similar pain and associated symptoms. Pain from the kidney is felt in the loin; pain from the ureter is felt in the loin, iliac fossa, groin or scrotum; pain from the bladder is felt suprapubically; pain from the bladder neck is referred to the perineum and down the urethra to the tip of the penis and pain from the prostate is felt variably in the perineum, rectum, groin, upper medial thigh, lower back or suprapubically. Associated symptoms may include fever, rigors (uncontrolled shaking), nausea or vomiting.

The complaint of a **lump** should also trigger a set of questions: its site, when and how was it first noticed, whether it is painful, whether it has changed in size, itched or bled, whether there have been previous similar lumps and any associated symptoms.

If the patient complains of LUTS, pneumaturia (indicative of colovesical fistula) haematuria, or abdominal pain / lump, a general inquiry should be made about altered bowel habit, appetite and weight loss.

The past medical and surgical history, drug history and allergies should be taken for all new patients. Certain drugs, including certain non-steroidal anti-inflammatory agents and cyclophosphamide, cause chronic cystitis and haematuria. In the social history, it is important to establish whether the patient lives with a responsible and caring adult, such as their spouse, who could help look after the patient after any operation that might be required. An enquiry about the patient's sexual activity status and/or sexual gender preferences may be relevant if there are genital or perineal symptoms. An obstetric history is important in female patients with voiding symptoms. A history of smoking is of concern with regards to bladder and kidney cancer. Alcohol intake may be relevant when considering frequency or nocturia. As regards the 'systems review', less detail is required than with a medical history.

The physical examination

General

The patient should be courteously invited to lie comfortably on their back with arms by their sides, on a couch in a warm private room. In so doing, their mobility in transferring from their chair (or wheelchair) to the couch is assessed and any help they require is noted. If the patient cannot lie comfortably because of a skeletal deformity or injury, examination must be carried out in an alternative position. If the patient cannot straighten one of his legs, or if it causes pain to do so, he may have psoas irritation due to a retroperitoneal abscess, mass or retrocaecal appendicitis. If the patient is female, a male doctor may wish to request the presence of a chaperone, or vice versa. The patient should be asked to expose his or her abdomen, groins and genitalia.

Inspection of the hands, face and neck and palpation of the radial pulse, cervical and supraclavicular areas are routine. Signs of any gross cardiovascular, respiratory, obesity or wasting disease are usually evident.

The abdomen

Observation

The abdomen is inspected and any asymmetry, distension or surface lesions (scars, skin lesions, sinuses) noted on a diagram together with other findings. The patient should be asked to point to the area of pain.

Palpation

The abdomen is palpated in the four anterior quadrants and in the two renal angles. During this, keep a close watch on the patient's face and eyes to detect **tenderness**, while causing the minimum of pain. Note any **mass**: assess its site, size, surface, consistency, mobility and tenderness. If it is in the loin, can it be palpated bimanually? Can you get above or below the lump? A **renal mass** is detected in the right or left upper quadrants; it may or may not be tender; only its lower margin is palpable and it may not be possible to get above it; the mass should be palpable bimanually unless it is too small; it should be slightly mobile downwards on inspiration. A **distended bladder** is palpable suprapubically as a dome-like mass (*Fig. 1.1*): this can be difficult

Fig. 1.1: This man presented with continuous dribbling incontinence. He had a firm non-tender lower abdominal swelling to just above the level of his umbilicus. It was not possible to 'get below' the swelling, which was dull to percussion. The diagnosis of chronic retention with overflow was made; upon urethral catheterization the residual urine volume was 2.8 l.

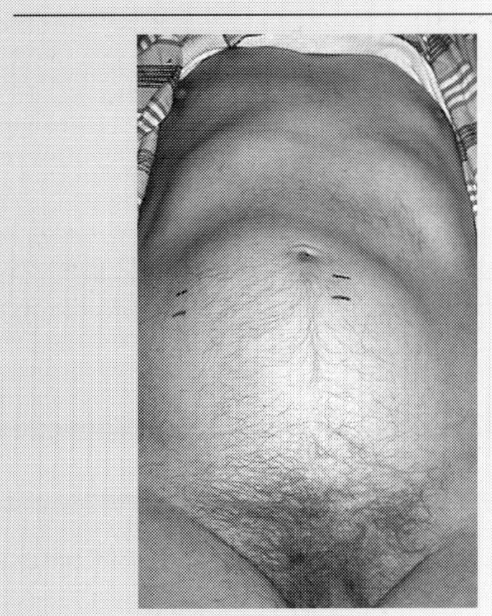

in obese patients. The palpable bladder may or may not be tender; it is not possible to get below it.

Percussion

A **renal mass** should be resonant to percussion (in theory) because, unlike the spleen or liver, it is a retroperitoneal structure, overlying which is gas-filled bowel. A **distended bladder** is dull to percussion, because it lifts the peritoneal contents away from the abdominal wall.

Auscultation

Not particularly helpful in the diagnosis of urological disease, but nevertheless an important part of the abdominal examination.

The groins and genitalia

Examination of the male groins and genitalia is discussed in Chapter 10. The patient should always be examined while watching the patient's face, lying and standing, so as not to hurt the patient or miss a hernia or varicocele. The foreskin, if present, should be retracted to ensure it is not tight and to reveal the glans penis. The urethral meatus is inspected to ensure it is in the normal position and is not scarred. The penile urethra and the corpora cavernosa are examined if the history suggests a relevance.

Examination of the female genitalia is done at the same time as a vaginal examination. This is not always necessary, but is indicated if the complaint relates to incontinence or other perineal symptoms. The ideal situation is with adequate light and the patient as relaxed as possible, lying in the left lateral position. A lubricated Simms speculum is inserted and the vaginal introitus is inspected for surface lesions or masses. The patient is asked to cough; any descent of the anterior or posterior vaginal walls or the cervix are noted; any urinary leakage is noted. If indicated, a bimanual vaginal examination is performed to palpate the cervix and adnexae (with the patient supine).

The digital rectal examination (DRE)

This is relevant for almost all male patients with urological complaints and some females with a combination of bladder, bowel or pelvic symptoms (*Fig. 1.2*). In Britain, the patient is examined in the left lateral position, though in the USA patients are examined in the knee–elbow position and in Italy the patient may be examined standing up! Whatever position, the patient must be reassured that the examination will be uncomfortable but quick. Patients with rectal stenosis, anal fissure, acute prostatitis, prostatic abscess or an inflammatory pelvic condition (diverticulitis, appendicitis, abscess, salpingitis) do find the DRE painful and this finding should be noted. The perianal skin and the anal sphincter are innervated by S2, 3 and 4. If neurological disease affecting the urinary sphincter is suspected, an assessment is made of perianal sensation and anal tone while performing a DRE. If either or both are reduced, then a lesion affecting these sacral nerves and indeed urinary sphincter function is highly likely.

Occasionally, a patient may be reluctant to undergo a DRE: in this case, he should be informed that it will not be possible to give an opinion on the state of his prostate or recommend any relevant treatment. Equally, the DRE may be avoided by doctors who are not confident of their findings: a recent survey of Oxford medical students sitting finals demonstrated that almost half had done five or fewer DREs and few felt confident in the interpretation of their findings. A business-like attitude and practical experience will resolve this lack of self-confidence. Further discussion is found in *Chapter 9*.

Fig. 1.2:
The DRE is important in the management of all patients complaining of urological, abdominal or bowel symptoms.

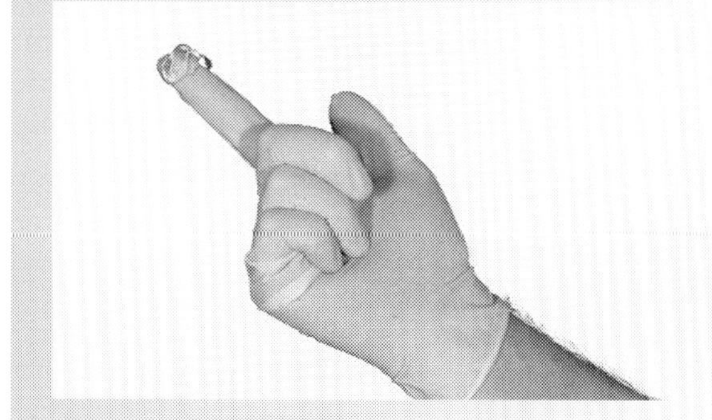

After the DRE, the patient should be cleaned and invited to dress for the remainder of the consultation, which will involve **discussion** regarding the differential diagnosis, proposed investigations or treatment, and perhaps prognosis.

Key points

- LUTS fall into filling (irritative) and voiding (obstructive) categories, concluding with an assessment of the 'bother' they are causing.
- Haematuria is painful or painless; initial, total or terminal. A good history may give a clue to the cause.
- Incontinence is generally categorized into four types: total, nocturnal, stress, urgency. Mixed stress and urgency may occur, particularly in multiparous women.
- The male groins and genitalia should always be examined with the patient lying and standing, while watching his face, so as not to miss a hernia or varicocele or hurt the patient.
- A painful DRE indicates likely rectal stenosis, anal fissure, acute prostatitis, prostatic abscess or a pelvic inflammatory condition.

Further reading

Browse N.L. (1997) *An Introduction to the Symptoms and Signs of Surgical Disease.* Third edition. Arnold, London.

CHAPTER 2

Urological investigations

Radiological investigations

The following are common radiological investigations used in urology. Many of these are discussed in the relevant chapters.

Renal ultrasound

This is quick, safe, inexpensive and non-invasive (*Fig. 2.1a*). It is suitable for detection of hydronephrosis, renal parenchymal tumours, renal cysts (*Fig. 2.1b*) and bladder tumours. Renal and bladder stones are usually detected, but pelvi-ureteric and ureteric stones are seldom seen. Post-micturition residual volume is calculated by measuring the dimensions of the bladder. Ultrasound is usually the recommended initial radiological examination of the kidneys for haematuria, but an IVU is indicated if the ultrasound and cystoscopy are normal.

Transrectal ultrasound (TRUS)

For defining the anatomy and volume of the prostate, and guiding prostatic biopsies. An uncomfortable investigation lasting 10 minutes, it is usually carried out as an outpatient investigation without anaesthetic. Antibiotic prophylaxis is administered to reduce the 1% risk of septicaemia following biopsy.

Scrotal ultrasound

For assessing masses and cysts of the testes, epididymes and spermatic cords. Ultrasound cannot exclude testicular torsion.

Intravenous urogram (IVU)

A plain X-ray incorporating kidneys, ureter and bladder (KUB) is taken as a 'control'. A contrast medium containing iodine is injected intravenously. Several radiographs are taken, firstly showing the uptake of contrast by the kidneys, seen as a nephrogram. Subsequent excretion of the contrast opacifies the pelvicalyceal systems and ureter, then fills the bladder (*Fig. 2.2*). Renal pelvicalyceal and ureteric anatomy and drainage should be seen,

Fig. 2.1: (a) A renal ultrasound showing a normal kidney in longitudinal section. The fat in the renal pelvis causes the high echogenicity; (b) a similar scan, showing a simple renal cyst (the lesion is circular, with an uncalcified wall and contains no internal echoes).

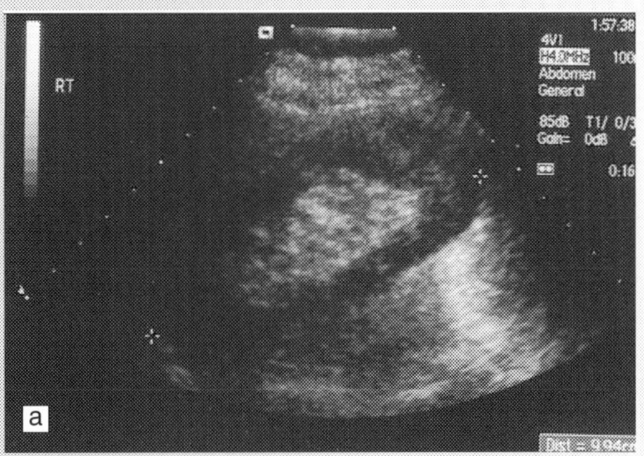

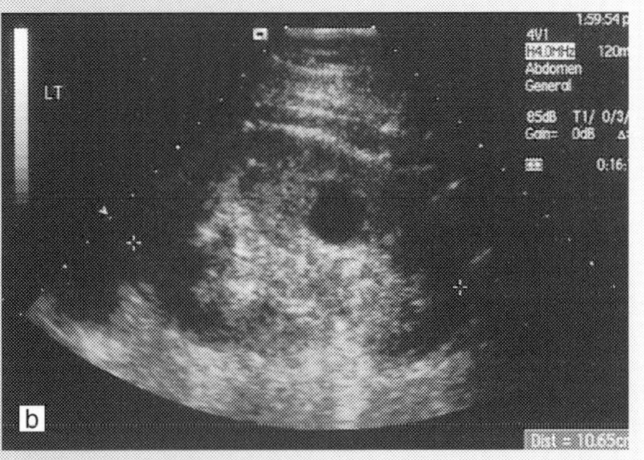

Fig. 2.2:
An IVU during the excretory phase. The large filling defect in the bladder was a transitional cell carcinoma.

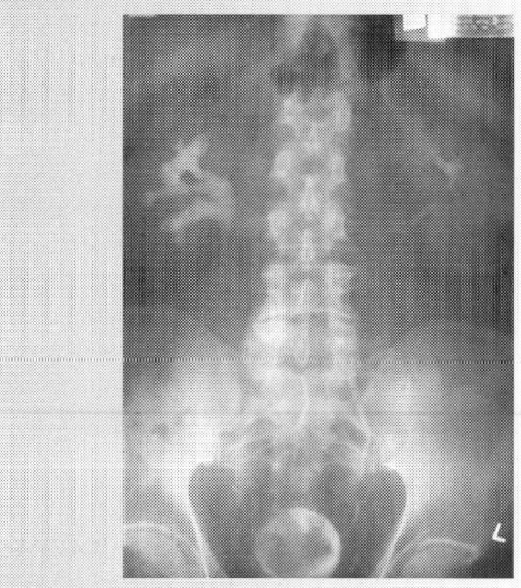

sometimes requiring a tomogram. Finally, a post-micturition X-ray gives a view of the distal ureter, or demonstrates poor emptying. Indications include haematuria, if the ultrasound and cystoscopy have failed to demonstrate any cause; renal or ureteric stone; recurrent urinary tract infections when the ultrasound is normal. Mild reactions to the injected contrast are common, including flushing and urticaria; severe allergic reactions, including facial swelling and cardiovascular collapse, are rare (1 per 100 000) with modern hypo-osmolar contrast media.

Urethrography and cystography

These investigations involve instillation of contrast into the urethra and/or bladder, followed by radiography. The contrast is usually introduced via a urethral catheter, but it can be introduced 'antegrade' through a suprapubic catheter. Indications for urethrography are to investigate urethral trauma or stricture disease. Indications for cystography are to investigate bladder trauma, to check for healing after reconstructive bladder surgery and to assess for ureteric reflux by asking the patient to void urine while a radiograph is taken (micturating cystourethrogram).

Computerized tomography (CT) urography

This is a sophisticated X-ray investigation, used for staging renal, bladder, retroperitoneal and testicular cancers. CT is also useful for identifying renal and ureteric calculi and investigating loin pain.

Magnetic resonance imaging (MRI)

A sophisticated imaging modality, involving the movement of electrons in a magnetic field, not X-rays. In urology, MRI is useful for staging prostate cancer, imaging renal cancer in the inferior vena cava and searching for intra-abdominal testicles.

Renography

A nuclear medicine study, involving intravenous administration of a Technetium^{99}-labelled substance which is taken up by the kidneys. The result is obtained using a gamma camera, counting the radioactivity over the kidneys and bladder. Renography is designed to investigate renal tubular function and excretion. **Static renography** (e.g. dimercapto-succinic acid [DMSA]) is useful for assessing relative renal function and scarring. The isotope is taken up by the proximal convoluted tubules but not excreted into the urine. **Dynamic renography** (e.g. mercaptoacetyl-triglycyl [MAG3]) is designed to assess whether hydronephrosis is caused by obstruction or whether the renal pelvis is capacious but not obstructed. The isotope is taken up by the tubules and then excreted into the urine; in the non-obstructed kidney, the isotope passes quickly down to the bladder (*Fig. 2.3*). However, in the presence of obstruction, the isotope activity is retained in the kidney. Intravenous frusemide during the study may help demonstrate obstruction by causing a diuresis.

Bone scan

Bone scanning is used for detecting bone metastases during staging of urological cancers. A technetium-labelled tracer is administered intravenously which is incorporated into bone. Scintigraphy is performed 3 hours later using a gamma camera (*Fig. 2.4*). False negative results may occur if metastases are osteolytic and false positive results may occur in the presence of Paget's disease

Fig. 2.3:
A normal dynamic renogram, indicating equal split renal function and no delay in uptake or excretion of isotope by either kidney (left-hand graph).

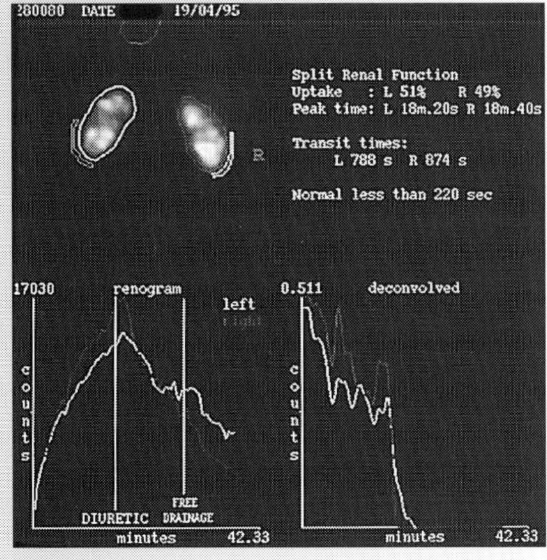

or osteoarthritis. Bone scanning is not as sensitive as an MRI bone marrow screen for the detection of bone metastases (*Fig. 2.5*).

Retrograde ureteropyelography

A ureteric catheter is passed up through the ureteric orifice using a cystoscope, under local or general anaesthetic. Contrast media is injected and radiographs are taken, giving superb views of the ureter, pelvi-ureteric junction and renal pelvicalyceal system. The site of filling defects or obstructing lesions is well seen (*Fig. 2.6*). Indications are for upper urinary tract obstruction or haematuria when poor views are obtained on IVU because of poor renal function or bowel gas, or the patient has a history of contrast allergy.

Antegrade ureteropyelography

Contrast media is injected via a percutaneous nephrostomy fine needle or tube, placed under local anaesthetic. Radiographs are taken, giving superb views of the pelvicalyceal system, pelvi-

Fig. 2.4:
A bone scan revealing several areas of abnormal uptake as 'hotspots', likely to represent bone metastases.

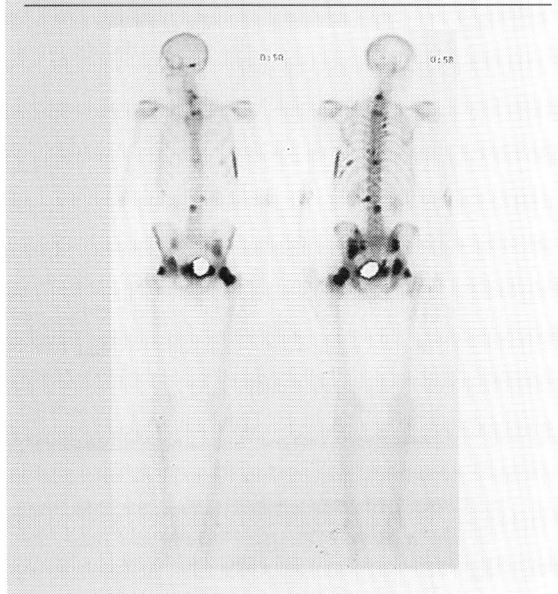

Fig. 2.5:
A coronal MRI of the spine and upper femora, demonstrating abnormal signal in L3 and one femur (the dark areas), likely to represent bone metastases.

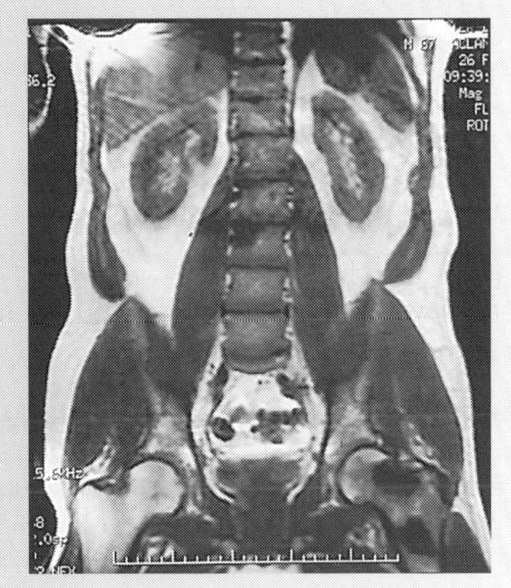

Fig. 2.6:
A retrograde ureteropyelogram, showing failure to fill the upper pole calyces, caused by a transitional cell carcinoma.

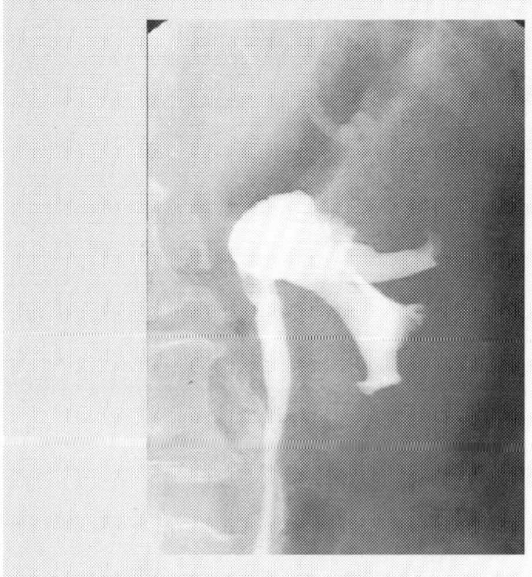

Fig. 2.7:
A vasogram, showing contrast media in the vas, seminal vesicle, ejaculatory duct and refluxing into the bladder via the prostatic urethra.

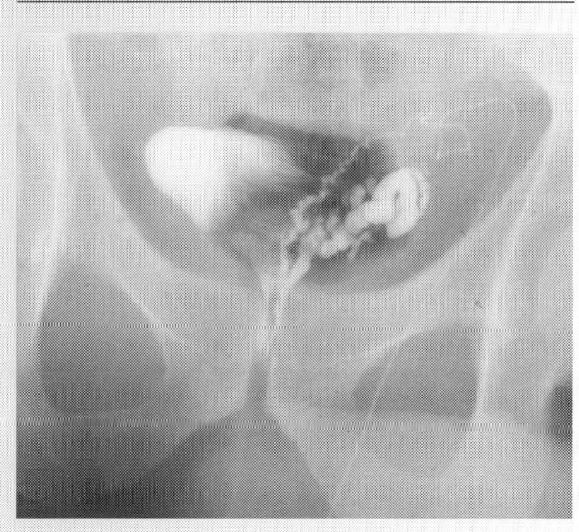

ureteric junction, ureter and bladder. The site of filling defects or obstructing lesions is well seen. Indications are for upper urinary tract obstruction or haematuria when retrograde ureterography is not possible, or the patient has an indwelling percutaneous nephrostomy tube.

Vasography

A fine cannula is placed in the lumen of each vas deferens at scrotal exploration. Radiological contrast is injected into each vas and radiograms taken. These demonstrate the vasa, seminal vesicle, ejaculatory ducts, prostatic urethra (*Fig. 2.7*). The level of any vasal obstruction is demonstrated. The main indication is male infertility with azospermia but normal hormone profile (see Chapter 10).

Angiography

This is demonstration of either arterial or venous anatomy by intravascular injection of contrast media, usually via a catheter introduced into the femoral artery. This is followed by a series of high-speed radiographs, made clearer by digital subtraction of other tissues (DSA). The renal arteriogram is most frequently requested in urology. An arterial phase delineates the anatomy of the renal artery or arteries, followed by a capillary blush and finally a venous phase shows the renal vein (*Fig. 2.8*). Indications include severe haematuria when other investigations have failed to demonstrate a cause, in case there is an arteriovenous malformation bleeding within the kidney, and as work-up prior to transplantation, partial nephrectomy or surgery on a horseshoe kidney.

Non-radiological investigations

Urine

The most basic investigation in urology is a **stick-test** of the urine (urinalysis). This is a quick, easy and cheap test carried out for every new patient attending the urology clinic, sometimes eliminating the need for more expensive investigations. Stick-tests, also known as reagent strips, demonstrate the presence of haemoglobin, leucocyte esterase (present with pyuria), nitrites (present with bacterial infection), protein (present with glomerular disease or infection) and glucose (present in poorly controlled and undiagnosed diabetics). False positive reactions to blood include

Fig. 2.8:
A renal arteriogram, performed after an IVU. It shows the arterial phase, with abnormal vasculature in the upper pole due to the presence of a renal carcinoma. The excretory phase of the IVU is apparent.

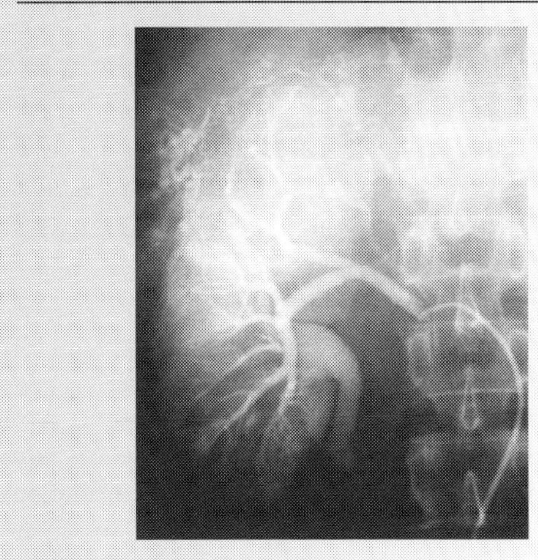

the presence of iodine and the antiseptic hypochlorite. Vitamin C may cause a false negative test for blood.

In the presence of a positive stick-test for leucocytes, nitrites or protein, a mid-stream urine (MSU) should be sent for **microscopy**, **culture** and **sensitivities**. A result indicating leucocytes but no bacterial growth indicates either a partially treated infection, or a sterile pyuria. The latter should prompt consideration of urinary tract tuberculosis, traditionally investigated by sending three **early morning urine** (EMU) samples for microscopy with Ziehl–Neelsen staining and Löwenstein–Jensen cultures. These take 6–9 weeks to complete. An MSU result indicating a mixed bacterial growth but no leucocytes should be considered contaminated by perineal flora, and repeated. A pure growth of 10^{4-5} colonies ml^{-1} in the presence of pyuria indicates urinary tract infection (UTI), and should be treated (see Chapter 7). The ova of *Schistosoma haematobium*, with their characteristic terminal spine, may be seen at microscopy.

Urine cytology is requested for patients with haematuria if the cause is not obvious on imaging and cystoscopy. Cytology is also helpful when following-up patients with carcinoma in-situ of the bladder. A fresh urine is stained with Papanicolaou stain and examined for the presence of malignant cells (characterized by abnormal nuclei and poor intercellular adhesion). False positive or 'suspicious' results may be caused by infection/inflammation; false negative results may occur in the presence of well-differentiated transitional carcinomas.

The Stamey **3-urine test** for bacterial prostatitis: an initial-void urine (V1), an MSU (V2) and urine following a prostatic massage (V3) are obtained. These are sent for culture: if V3 contains bacteria while V1 and V2 do not, the diagnosis of prostatitis is clinched. Any other combination of results does not! This procedure is time-consuming but helpful in selected cases.

24-hour urine collections: calcium, citrate, oxalate, creatinine clearance: see Chapter 8.

Semen analysis

Usually requested (twice) for men complaining of infertility. Fresh ejaculates are examined microscopically. Sperm density, motility, morphology and forward progression are assessed (see Chapter 10). Semen culture or cytology are rarely helpful in the management of any complaint.

Blood tests

Prostate-specific antigen: see Chapter 9.

Creatinine and electrolytes.

Alpha-fetoprotein, human chorionic gonadotrophin, lactate dehydrogenase: see Chapter 9.

Follicular stimulating hormone (FSH), luteinizing hormone (LH), testosterone: see Chapter 10.

Calcium, urate: see Chapter 8.

Cystourethroscopy

This is visual inspection of the inside of the urethra and bladder. It is indicated for patients with stick-test, microscopic or macroscopic haematuria, recurrent urinary tract infections, unexplained voiding symptoms or surveillance of patients with a history of bladder cancer. Cystourethroscopy can be undertaken either under local anaesthetic using a flexible cystoscope, or under general anaesthesia using a rigid instrument. Most patients will have the former, although the capacity for biopsy is limited.

Rigid cystoscopy is better for young or anxious patients and those in whom there is a high likelihood of detecting a lesion requiring resection.

Flexible ureterorenoscopy

Tiny flexible endoscopes now exist, which can be introduced transurethrally into the ureter and passed to the renal pelvis, usually under sedational anaesthesia. This is indicated for visualization of ureteric or renal pelvic lesions, although the capacity for biopsy is limited due to the size of the instruments. The rigid ureteroscope is more widely used, requiring general anaesthesia.

Urodynamic studies

A range of investigations, designed to assess bladder behaviour. Further detail is provided in Chapter 4.

Frequency/volume charts

These are indicated for patients who complain of urinary frequency. The patient measures the volume of each void and records the time on a chart, for seven consecutive days. The total fluid intake volume is also estimated for each day. The information gained can be very useful. For example, if the patient is passing large quantities of urine frequently, she should be investigated for diabetes mellitus and insipidus. Another patient might be voiding more than one third of his total output overnight, indicating a degree of cardiac failure.

The flow rate

This is a measurement of urine flow velocity, in millilitres per second, with time. Usually three tests are indicated for men (and occasionally women) with lower urinary tract symptoms (LUTS) to determine whether they are likely to have bladder outflow obstruction (BOO). The patient waits until he has a full bladder, then passes urine into the flowmeter and a flow curve is obtained, indicating the volume voided, the time taken and the maximum flow rate (Q_{max}). A normal Q_{max} is >20 ml s^{-1}. The majority of men whose Q_{max} is <15 ml s^{-1} have BOO. A few men whose Q_{max} is >15 ml s^{-1} have BOO and a few men whose Q_{max} is <15 ml s^{-1} do not have BOO, but a weak bladder (detrusor failure). *Figures 2.9, 2.10* and *2.11* illustrate examples of flow rates and residual volume measurements.

Pressure–flow studies

More invasive, this study, properly known as a **cystometrogram**, involves inserting rectal and bladder catheters and measuring the pressures when the bladder is filling and voiding. This study is indicated for patients with urgency who may have unstable contractions, or LUTS in whom flow rates and postmicturition residual volumes are equivocal for BOO. It is done as an outpatient procedure using local anaesthetic. Pressure–flow studies can be combined with fluoroscopic screening, termed **videocystometrography** (VCMG) to obtain a visual record of the bladder, ureters and urethra as well as the pressures during filling and voiding. This sophisticated investigation is indicated for patients with incontinence or neurological disease affecting their bladders (see Chapters 5 and 6).

Fig. 2.9:
A poor flow rate (Q_{max} 3 ml s^{-1}) with a residual volume of 1847 ml (please note!) indicating severe bladder outflow obstruction.

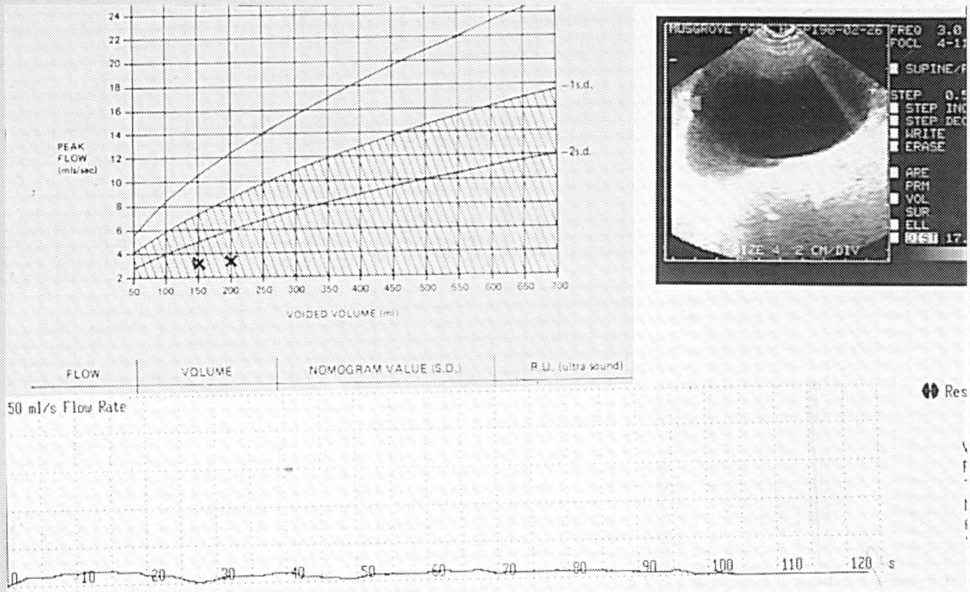

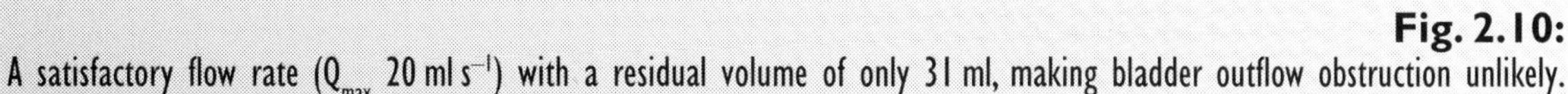

Fig. 2.10:
A satisfactory flow rate (Q_{max} 20 ml s^{-1}) with a residual volume of only 31 ml, making bladder outflow obstruction unlikely.

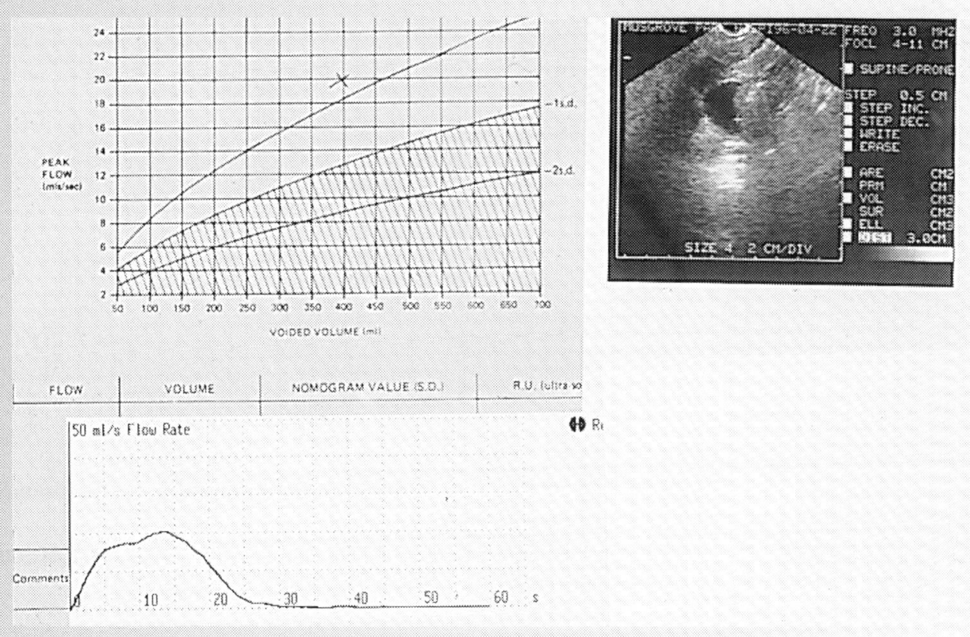

Fig. 2.11:
A prolonged flow rate (Q_{max} 10 ml s^{-1}) and a residual volume calculated at 101 ml, indicating likely prostatic bladder outflow obstruction.

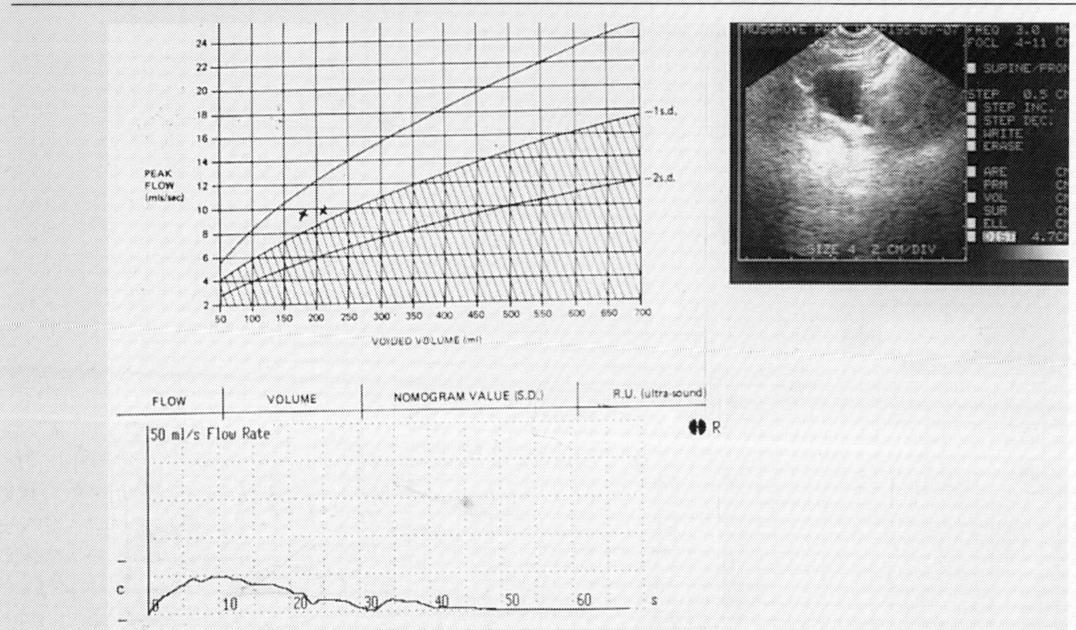

Key points

- Urinalysis using the urine stick-test is quick, easy and inexpensive. It is carried out for every new patient attending the urology clinic, sometimes eliminating the need for more expensive urine investigations.
- The complaint of haematuria warrants a renal ultrasound and a cystoscopy. If they are normal, an IVU may detect an abnormality in the pelvicalyceal system or ureter, not detected by ultrasound.
- If requested to comment upon an IVU, always ask to see the control film first, since a staghorn renal calculus may look like contrast in the pelvicalyceal system.
- Dynamic renography is the gold standard investigation to demonstrate pelviureteric junction obstruction.
- Urinary flow rate and residual volume provide a guide to the presence of bladder outflow obstruction, but a pressure–flow urodynamic study provides proof and is considered the gold standard.

CHAPTER 3

Urological emergencies and trauma

Urinary retention

Urinary retention is, simply, the inability to empty the bladder. There are several types of retention, and each requires different management. Urinary retention is very uncommon in women.

Complete and painful inability to empty the bladder where the bladder is catheterized and less than 800 ml of urine is drained is called **acute urinary retention**. Complete and painful inability to empty the bladder where the bladder is catheterized and >800 ml of urine is drained is called **acute-on-chronic urinary retention**. There is a situation where the patient is still able to void, but because they are unable to completely empty their bladder and after each void they consistently leave >500 ml of urine behind, they are said to be in **chronic retention**. This is a somewhat empirical definition of chronic retention, and others define chronic retention as a post-void residual urine volume of >300 ml, but the point is that patients with chronic retention of urine retain a **substantial** volume of urine in their bladders after each void.

The various forms of chronic retention of urine (be they acute-on-chronic or simply chronic) may be associated with such large volumes of retained urine and such high bladder pressures that patients develop back-pressure on their kidneys, leading to the appearances on ultrasound scanning of hydronephrosis and the presence of a raised serum creatinine (which falls, over the course of several days, after catheterization). Such forms of chronic retention are called **high pressure acute-on-chronic retention** and **high pressure chronic retention**. Patients with chronic retention, but no hydronephrosis are said to have **low pressure chronic retention**.

Why all the fuss about retention volume? Are these definitions necessary?

Firstly, without recording the volume of urine drained from the bladder you cannot make a diagnosis of urinary retention. Some patients present with a history of lower abdominal pain and failing to pass urine (or passing only very small quantities), and have suprapubic tenderness or a tender lower abdominal mass, all of which is suggestive of acute urinary retention. However, when they are catheterized, their bladder is empty or contains only a low volume of urine (well below 800 ml). They are clearly not in urinary retention and there is some other cause for their pain and tenderness such as perforated or ischaemic bowel. They are fluid depleted, hence the history of not passing any urine. So, recording urine volume in a case of suspected urinary retention allows you to confirm the diagnosis. You should record this in the notes so other clinicians looking after the patient know that you made the correct diagnosis.

Secondly, retention volume is useful for determining subsequent management and it also has prognostic value. A patient with high-pressure chronic retention is likely to have a diuresis once the obstruction has been relieved by passage of a catheter. Recording retention volume allows you to anticipate this diuresis and allows you to be aware of the potential risk of postural hypotension. The diuresis can be profound, many litres of urine being produced in the first few days. The diuresis is due to:

(a) off-loading of retained salt and water (retained in the weeks prior to the episode of retention);
(b) dissipation of the corticomedullary concentration gradient caused by reduced urinary flow through the loop of Henle with maintenance of blood flow through the chronically obstructed kidney;
(c) an osmotic diuresis caused by the high urea level that occurs in such patients.

The diuresis does not usually cause any problems and it usually resolves spontaneously within a matter of days. It is said to be physiological (rather than pathological) because it represents a normal diuretic response to fluid overload. Rarely the patient may develop symptomatic postural hypotension (a preceding postural drop in blood pressure can provide some warning of this) and in such cases intravenous fluid replacement may be necessary.

Retention volume can also be used to indicate the need for subsequent prostate surgery (transurethral resection of the prostate – TURP). Patients with large retention volumes (>1000 ml) are less likely than those with smaller volumes to void spontaneously after a trial of catheter removal, and although it is always nice to give them the benefit of the doubt, it is useful to be able to predict that subsequent TURP is likely. A substantial proportion of patients who undergo TURP for urinary retention will not void when their catheter is removed a few days post-operatively. Those with acute retention have a 10% risk of failure to void and those with chronic and acute-on-chronic retention have a 38% and 44% chance of failure to void after surgery. A total of 99% eventually void successfully on subsequent catheter removal several weeks later (Reynard and Shearer, 1999). Thus, retention volume predicts the likelihood of failure to void in these cases. This allows the patient to be counselled pre-operatively about their likelihood of voiding after the operation. It is also reassuring for the surgeon to know that failure to void after TURP is not a complication, but a normal event in the post-operative recovery of many patients.

Suprapubic catheterization

Most patients with urinary retention will initially be managed by insertion of a urethral catheter. However, in some cases it may not be possible to pass a urethral catheter and a suprapubic catheter should then be placed. This may be undertaken using a percutaneous trocar introducer under local anaesthetic. This should be a reasonably large catheter (a 12 or 14 Ch catheter). Smaller catheters will block within a matter of weeks and cannot easily be replaced, whereas a larger bore catheter is less likely to block and much easier to replace, once the suprapubic catheter track has matured.

There are certain golden rules and contraindications to consider. These are designed to establish that the tender suprapubic mass you can feel is the bladder and not bowel or an abdominal aortic aneurysm (AAA)! It is generally taken that the presence of a lower midline abdominal incision is a contraindication to suprapubic catheter placement because adhesions may cause a segment of bowel to be closely applied to the internal surface of the incision. The golden rules are: first, palpate and percuss the bladder, making sure it is not pulsatile; second, aspirate urine with a fine needle. If you cannot aspirate urine, **abandon the procedure**. When it has not been possible to aspirate urine suprapubically, or when there is a lower midline abdominal incision there may be loops of adherent bowel, ultrasound-guided placement of a suprapubic catheter or open suprapubic catheter placement under direct vision in an operating theatre should be carried out.

Clot retention

This type of retention can occur as a result of bleeding from a renal or bladder tumour or, commonly, following TURP. It is rare for the patient, even with seemingly very heavy haematuria, to have lost so much blood that they become haemodynamically unstable or require blood transfusion, but as with blood loss from any site it is a wise precaution to insert a wide bore intravenous line and to at least group and save the patient's serum, as well as measuring baseline haemoglobin, platelets and blood clotting. Anticoagulant and antiplatelet drugs should be stopped, if feasible.

The acute management of a patient who tells you that they have been passing blood in their urine and was then unable to void involves insertion of a 3-way 'haematuria' catheter. These come in various sizes, but a 22 or 24 Ch catheter will allow you to evacuate clot and irrigate the bladder (*Fig. 3.1*). Haematuria catheters have a large distal eye hole, which allows relatively large clots to be aspirated from the bladder. Usually, following aspiration of clot and bladder irrigation, the haematuria settles down and the patient may then undergo upper tract imaging (an IVU or ultrasound) and later a flexible cystoscopy. It is customary to perform cystoscopy after the bleeding has settled down and the catheter has been removed,

Fig. 3.1:
A Rusch 3-way haematuria catheter – note the large distal eye hole which allows clots to be evacuated.

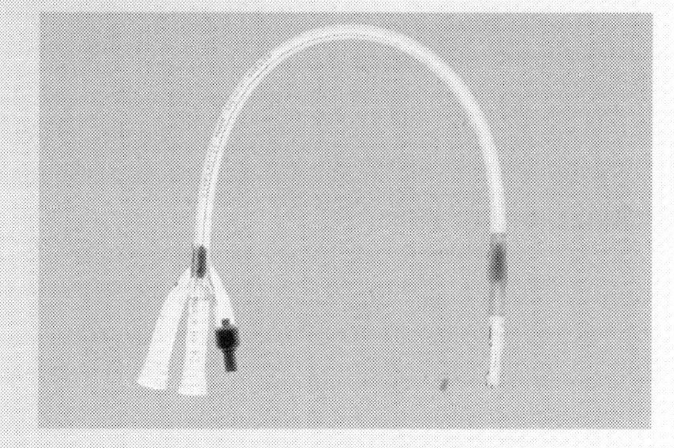

firstly because visualization of the bladder will not be obscured by the presence of blood, and secondly because the mucosal oedema caused by the catheter will have resolved. However, if the bleeding does not resolve with simple bladder irrigation, and assuming the source is thought to be from the bladder or prostate (i.e. upper tract imaging is normal) then the patient may require cystoscopy under anaesthesia to identify and treat the cause.

Ureteric colic

Ureteric colic is caused by the passage of a stone, but occasionally by a clot and rarely a necrosed renal papilla, from the kidney through the ureter. The combination of local inflammation and a stretched collecting system and ureter contracting and trying to eject the stone classically causes sudden onset of loin pain, which is very severe and colicky in nature. It may not entirely disappear between exacerbations. Macroscopic or microscopic haematuria may occur, though in a small proportion of cases it may be absent. Though most patients with ureteric colic are young or middle-aged, it can occur in children and elderly individuals. While one should consider other potential diagnoses in a patient of any age, this is particularly important in the elderly where the list of differentials is wider.

A total of 50% of cases of suspected ureteric colic have normal imaging studies or demonstrate another cause for the pain. The list of differential diagnoses includes leaking AAA, perforated peptic ulcer, inflammatory bowel conditions, testicular torsion, ruptured ectopic pregnancy in women, acute appendicitis and myocardial infarction. While a careful history and examination may help in identifying the exact cause of the pain, a high index of suspicion for these alternative diagnoses must be maintained, particularly in elderly patients who are more likely to have other bowel and vascular disease.

Investigations

IVU is the mainstay of imaging in cases of suspected renal colic in most hospitals. However, some centres prefer to use CTU (CT urography) (*Fig. 3.2*). This allows more rapid urinary tract imaging without the need for contrast injection and has a high sensitivity for ureteric stones. In cases where no ureteric stone is identified, CTU has the advantage over IVU of demonstrating other intra-abdominal pathology. There is a trend towards CTU replacing IVU in the diagnosis of loin pain.

Treatment

Analgesia: the non-steroidal anti-inflammatory drug diclofenac can provide very effective relief of pain, though opiates (usually pethidine) may also

Fig. 3.2:
A CT urogram showing a right ureteric stone at the vesico-ureteric junction.

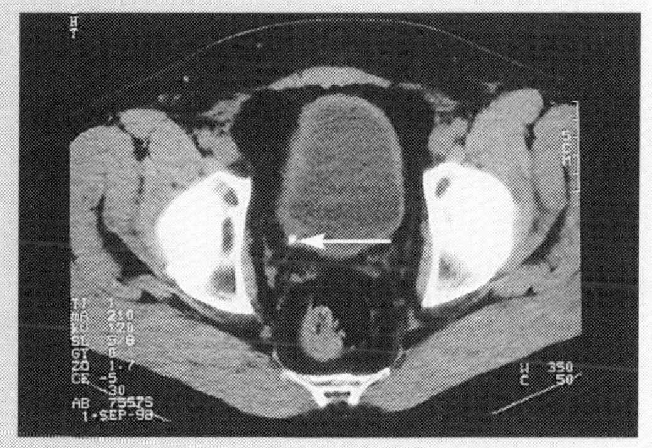

be required. In most cases of ureteric stones the pain will usually resolve spontaneously, either as a result of passage of the stone out of the ureter or once it has come to a halt somewhere in the ureter. Persistent pain (for more than a few days) is an indication for relief of obstruction, either by insertion of a percutaneous nephrostomy into the kidney or by the retrograde passage of a double J stent from bladder to ureter. An alternative, available in some hospitals, is ureteroscopic stone extraction.

Management of stones which fail to pass spontaneously is discussed in Chapter 8.

The obstructed, infected kidney

There are instances where a patient presents with a ureteric stone and certain features lead you to suspect that there is associated urinary infection. The scenario of ureteric obstruction combined with infection can rapidly (within hours) lead to damage to the affected kidney with long term scarring and loss of functioning renal tissue. Furthermore, infection in an obstructed kidney can lead on to the development of pyonephrosis (pus in the kidney) or a renal or perirenal abscess. Again, this will result in serious damage to the kidney.

Diagnosis

The diagnosis of infection in an obstructed kidney is essentially a clinical one, based on the presence of a **fever** in a patient with radiologic evidence of obstruction. An IVU (or CT) will confirm the presence of a ureteric stone. Alternatively the presence of an obstructed, infected ureteric stone may be suspected in a patient with ultrasonographic evidence of hydronephrosis and a fever. Bacteria are not necessarily seen in the urine nor grown on culture if the obstructing stone prevents passage of bacteria into the bladder.

Treatment

Resuscitation with intravenous fluids, analgesia, intravenous broad-spectrum antibiotics (e.g. gentamicin combined with ampicillin) and most importantly drainage of the pus with relief of obstruction by percutaneous nephrostomy or retrograde ureteric stent insertion.

Septic shock

Septic shock is a combination of sepsicaemia with hypotension. Sepsicaemia is the syndrome of clinical evidence of infection by which we mean tachycardia (pulse >90 min^{-1}), tachypnoea (>20 respirations min^{-1}), hyperthermia (core temperature >38.3°C; though occasionally hypothermia – core temperature <35.6°C may occur), and evidence of inadequate tissue perfusion such as hypoxia, oliguria and elevated plasma lactic acid levels. Hypotension is defined as a systolic blood pressure <90 mmHg.

Septic shock is traditionally thought of as being due to Gram-negative organisms, but it may also be due to Gram-positive bacteria and fungi. However, in the context of urologic surgery and manipulation of the urinary tract, Gram-negative organisms (e.g. *E. coli*, *Klebsiella*, *Enterobacter serratia*, *Proteus*, *Pseudomonas*) are the commonest bacteria to be isolated.

Several factors are involved in the pathophysiology of septic shock. The lipopolysaccharide layer of Gram-negative bacterial cell walls (known as endotoxin) activates humoral pathways (e.g. complement, bradykinin, the coagulation system), macrophages and other cells involved in mediating inflammation. The lipid A part of the lipopolysaccharide is thought to be responsible for most of the toxicity of the endotoxin molecule. Exotoxins (e.g. exotoxin A produced by *Ps. aeruginosa*) can also initiate septic shock.

Common urological procedures which may be followed by septic shock include TURP, and ureteroscopic and percutaneous stone removal, but even simple catheterization, particularly in the presence of infected urine, can be responsible. Septic shock may occur even when pre-operative urine cultures show no significant growth of bacteria and this forms the basis for the use of prophylactic antibiotics in all patients undergoing TURP and stone surgery irrespective of whether they have an MSU positive for bacteria or not.

Subsequent management of suspected septic shock includes culture of urine, blood and any drain fluid, appropriate antibiotics, volume expansion with normal saline or a plasma expander and oxygen. Monitoring of vital functions should be performed and this should also include measurement of urine output (catheterization allows this to be measured accurately) and blood gases.

Anuria and bilateral ureteric obstruction

Patients who present with anuria (passing no urine at all or very small volumes) and who have bilateral hydronephrosis on ultrasound scanning usually have bilateral ureteric obstruction, due either to bladder outlet obstruction, locally invasive prostate cancer, invasive bladder tumours involving both ureteric orifices within the bladder or some retroperitoneal obstructing condition such as malignant retroperitoneal lymphadenopathy (of which there are many causes) or retroperitoneal fibrosis. If the bladder is empty on ultrasound or catheterization and the kidneys are hydronephrotic, then the obstruction is above the level of the bladder outlet. This will be the case, for example, when a prostate cancer invades the lower ureters.

Diagnosis

History and, in particular, examination are often enough to make the diagnosis, which may then be confirmed by further investigations. Thus, a patient with a history of recurrent haematuria preceding their anuria by some months may well have a bladder cancer. Back pain suggests retroperitoneal lymphadenopathy. Digital rectal examination of the prostate in males and pelvic examination in females is crucial and may suggest the presence of a locally invasive prostate or cervical cancer. Supraclavicular, cervical or axillary lymphadenopathy may provide an easy target for histological confirmation by biopsy of whatever malignant process is causing the retroperitoneal lymphadenopathy (this can occur from as far afield as the breast or lung!).

Investigations

Measurement of serum potassium, urea and creatinine are important. If prostate cancer is suspected serum PSA should be measured. A chest X-ray may show evidence of metastatic or primary malignant disease in the lungs. Abdominal and pelvic CT will confirm the presence of retroperitoneal or pelvic lymphadenopathy. Transrectal ultrasound and prostatic biopsy are used to provide histological evidence of prostate cancer and cystoscopy will diagnose a bladder cancer.

Treatment

As for unilateral renal obstruction the mainstay of acute treatment is relief of the obstruction, by percutaneous nephrostomies or retrograde ureteric stents. If the obstruction is distal in the ureter, it is often impossible to pass a stent across the obstruction from below.

Fournier's gangrene

This is a necrotizing fasciitis of the male genitalia. It has an abrupt onset and is a rapidly fulminating gangrene which results in destruction of the genitalia. Multiple organisms may be cultured from the infected tissue, both aerobic (e.g. *E. coli*, *Klebsiella*, enterococci) and anaerobic (*Bacteroides*, *Clostridium*, *Fusobacterium*, microaerophilic streptococci). It is believed that there is aerobic–anaerobic synergy between the aerobic and anaerobic organisms (i.e. the organisms promote growth and division of each other). Several conditions are thought to predispose to Fournier's gangrene, including diabetes, local trauma (which may be minor), paraphimosis, extravasation of urine from the urethra (e.g. due to traumatic catheterization), circumcision and perianal surgery or sepsis.

The necrotizing fasciitis usually starts as an area of cellulitis adjacent to an entry wound on the penis, scrotum or perineum. This rapidly progresses to a painful, erythematous area which is tender to touch and as the infection progresses subcutaneous gas may be palpated (a characteristic sensation of crepitus is felt when the skin is depressed). The lower abdominal wall may be involved. Rapid onset of gangrene of the skin and subcutaneous tissues of the perineum, shaft of the penis and scrotum follows (*Fig. 3.3*). The patient is systemically very unwell and if treatment is not instituted immediately death may ensue.

The mainstays of treatment are high-dose intravenous antibiotics with a spectrum of activity against aerobes, anaerobes, Gram-positive and Gram-negative organisms. An initial regime of ampicillin, gentamicin and metronidazole is appropriate until sensitivities from blood or tissue

Fig. 3.3:
A case of Fournier's gangrene. Note the penile swelling and developing blisters (bullae).

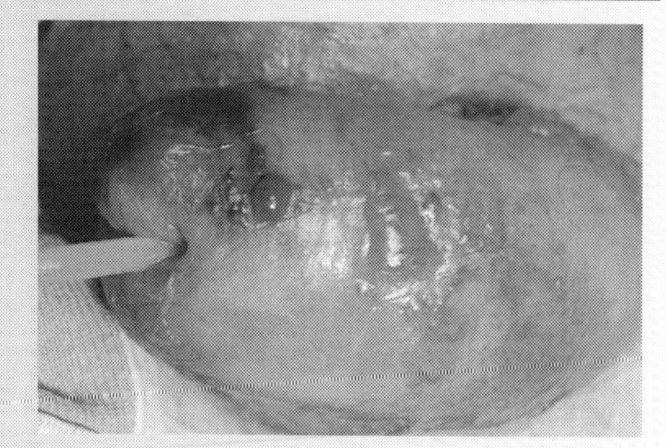

culture are available. Surgical debridement should accompany this regime of antibiotics and this should be done without delay. Obviously necrotic tissue (skin and fascia) together with a margin of apparently healthy surrounding tissue should be removed. This may involve the removal of large areas of tissue and later skin grafting may be required (if the patient survives). Hyperbaric oxygen treatment has been used and is thought to reduce mortality (though not surprisingly there are no randomized, controlled studies comparing one treatment against another) (Dahm et al., 2000). Insertion of a suprapubic catheter may be required to divert urine from the urethra if extravasation of urine from the urethra has occurred. Mortality is in the range of 10–50%.

Torsion of the testis

During fetal development the entire testis may become enveloped by the visceral layer of peritoneum in its descent into the scrotum, and this results in a so-called bell-clapper testis, which can easily rotate on its pedicle and so occlude its blood supply. A urological emergency, the testis is rotated about its intravaginal cord, rendering it ischaemic, swollen and painful. Undescended testes are particularly prone to torsion in the inguinal canal. Although it can occur at any age, the commonest age for torsion is 10–16 years and is uncommon over 30 years.

Presentation

Severe scrotal pain of acute onset, radiating to the groin and sometimes to the iliac fossa and to the renal area, reflecting the origin of the developing testis from the region of the kidney. Very occasionally the pain in the loin may be more severe than the scrotal pain, and a mistaken diagnosis of ureteric colic is made, for the want of not examining the testicle (which will be very tender on palpation). There may be associated vomiting. Fever can occur if the presentation is delayed. Urinary symptoms are absent. Some patients have a history of similar pain that resolved spontaneously, suggesting **intermittent torsion**. On examination, the patient is usually in considerable distress with pain. Pyrexia is uncommon unless presentation is late and the testis is necrotic. The groins look normal, though there may be tenderness (without peritonism) in the iliac fossa and groin on the affected side. The scrotum is usually swollen and discoloured red/blue. The testis may be seen to lie high and transversely in the scrotum, compared with the normal testis. It is swollen and very tender to touch, often too tender to examine properly. Urinalysis is negative.

Differential diagnosis

The differential diagnoses are principally epididymitis, and torsion of an appendix testis or appendix epididymis. Careful clinical examination which elicits tenderness and swelling in the epididymis, and a completely non-tender testis suggests a diagnosis of epididymitis. However, if there is any testicular tenderness it is safest to explore the scrotum to exclude or confirm the presence of torsion (see Chapter 7). It must be remembered that when the testis twists, not only is the blood supply to the testis occluded, but so too is that to the epididymis, and the tenderness in the epididymis may therefore be due to torsion.

Treatment

Adequate **analgesia**, for example intramuscular pethidine, is essential. Once the diagnosis is made, or if there is any possibility of testicular torsion, **scrotal exploration** must be undertaken as soon as possible. Irreversible ischaemic changes occur after

6 hours of torsion. The testis is de-torted and **bilateral orchidopexy** performed using non-absorbable material to prevent future torsion on either side. If the testis is black and fails to recover after several minutes, **orchidectomy** is necessary (the patient should be warned and consented pre-operatively). There is evidence to suggest that the dead testis may elicit an immune reaction against the contralateral normal testis (as the blood–testis barrier which normally isolates the immunogenic spermatozoa from the rest of the body breaks down), and this may subsequently affect the hormonal and spermatogenic function of the opposite testis.

Sometimes it is possible to 'de-tort' the testis percutaneously, but this can be painful and orchidopexies are still required.

If there is a history of intermittent episodes of sudden-onset of scrotal pain in a young male, the diagnosis of intermittent torsion should be considered and prophylactic bilateral orchidopexies offered.

Torsion of the appendix testis and appendix epididymis

The appendix of the testis is the cranial remnant of the paramesonephric (Müllerian) duct. The appendix of the epididymis is the cranial remnant of the mesonephric (Wolffian) duct. Both tiny vestigial structures are located at the upper pole of the testis or epididymis, respectively and are pedunculated on short stalks.

These appendages can tort, mostly in childhood, producing symptoms and signs similar to those of testicular torsion. The patient is usually less distressed than one with testicular torsion. Other differences include the normal position of the testis, though the swelling and tenderness often obscure this, and the absence of iliac fossa tenderness. Sometimes, in cases presenting early, a 'blue dot' is visible through the scrotal wall at the upper pole of the testis. If the tenderness is localized to this, the diagnosis is made.

Treatment can be conservative if the diagnosis is certain, since the pain will often last only a few days and the testis is not affected. However, the majority require exploration because of diagnostic uncertainty. A torted appendage is excised and orchidopexies need not be performed.

Priapism

Priapism is a prolonged painful erection, not associated with sexual desire. After 3 hours the erection becomes increasingly painful, probably because of ischaemia and toxic metabolites. Priapism is classified into the common ischaemic acidotic 'low-flow' and the rare non-ischaemic 'high-flow' types (*Table 3.1*). The high-flow priapism is not painful, and is caused by the traumatic development of arteriocavernous fistulae.

Diagnosis and investigations

There is little to cause diagnostic confusion in this urological emergency. The cause of the priapism is usually evident from the history, presence of pain, the presence of coexistent disease (haematological, neurological, malignancy), drug history and history of perineal trauma. In young boys priapism is most often due to sickle cell disease or malignancy (e.g. leukaemia). In the older age group it may be idiopathic, but most commonly it is iatrogenic, caused by intracavernosal self-injection therapy used for ED (see Chapter 10), other drugs (e.g. antidepressants such as trazodone and fluoxetine; clozapine; chlorpromazine; alpha-adrenergic blockers), sickle-cell disease, malignancy (leukaemia, metastatic prostate cancer, renal cancer and melanoma) and neurologic disorders (spinal cord injury, cauda equina compression, intervertebral disc prolapse). It has also been reported to occur in association with total parenteral nutrition, particularly with the use of intravenous fat emulsions. This is a low-flow type priapism, thought to be due to increased

Table 3.1: Causes of priapism

High-flow	Low-flow
Perineal trauma	Iatrogenic: PGE1, trazodone
Penile trauma	Sickle cell disease
	Malignancy: leukaemia, prostate
	Neuropathies: spinal cord lesions
	Idiopathic: prolonged sexual activity

coagulability of the blood or to fat emboli. Perineal or penile trauma can lead to priapism, which may be low-flow (where the venous outflow of the penis is occluded by thrombosis or severe penile oedema) or high-flow (where the cavernosal artery ruptures leading to uncontrolled flow of arterial blood into the corpora). Perineal trauma can occur as a result of bicycle cross bar injuries – where a cyclist comes to a sudden halt and in doing so is thrown onto the cross-bar of his bicycle.

Examination will reveal a dusky erection involving only the corpora cavernosa, with flaccidity of the glans and corpus spongiosum.

Blood gas measurement on blood aspirated from the rigid corpora and duplex ultrasound scanning can be very helpful in determining what type of priapism is present.

Treatment

Low-flow type: Emergency treatment is required, because of the risk of irreversible ischaemic damage, resulting in corporal fibrosis if >6 hours has elapsed. Aspirating one of the corpora will decompress the priapism and relieve pain. This is accomplished using a wide-bore butterfly inserted perpendicularly to its full depth, aspirating until flaccidity is achieved, then waiting. Some priapisms require no further treatment. Others will re-develop, requiring further aspiration. It two aspirations fail, a tourniquet is applied to the penile base, further aspiration is carried out and a vasoconstrictor (e.g. 0.05–0.1 mg of adrenaline diluted in 5 ml saline) is injected and the tourniquet released after 5 minutes. The patient's blood pressure should be monitored after administration of these agents. Usually, this is successful. If the priapism returns, a shunt procedure is undertaken under anaesthetic. This involves creating a fistula from the corpora cavernosa to either the glans using a Tru-cut needle or to the corpus spongiosum or the saphenous vein.

Where a coexistent medical condition is likely to be the cause of the priapism then this should be treated in its on right, together with aspiration and irrigation of the corpora (as described above) if the priapism is of the low-flow variety. For example, in sickle cell disease with priapism (which is most usually of the low-flow type) the patient should receive analgesia, rehydration with intravenous fluids combined with alkalinization of plasma, oxygen should be administered and haemoglobin S levels should be measured. Exchange transfusion may be required to lower the concentration of sickling red cells which by occluding venous outflow from the penis contribute to the development of the priapism in sickle cell disease. Cases of malignant priapism should receive treatment specific to the condition.

High-flow type: less of an emergency and rare, a selective internal pudendal arteriogram is indicated to identify the fistula. Radiological embolization is usually successful in reducing flow through the fistula.

Urological trauma

Renal trauma

The kidneys are retroperitoneal structures. Their posterior abdominal location, combined with a thick surrounding layer of perirenal fat, the posterior abdominal wall muscles and the lower ribs posteriorly, protects them against injury. As a consequence renal injury usually requires considerable force and it is therefore not surprising that it is often associated with injuries to other intra-abdominal organs.

Presentation

Renal injuries are most often due to blunt trauma (road traffic accidents, falls, contact sports and assaults) and are less commonly caused by stabbing or gunshot wounds, so-called penetrating injuries. Penetrating injuries are proportionately more common in urban environments. From a management point of view, this classification system – blunt versus penetrating – is useful, because we know from large series of renal injuries that only 2% of blunt injuries will require surgical exploration for repair of the renal injury, whereas approximately 50% of penetrating injuries will do so. Furthermore, we also know that the great majority of patients with gun-shot wounds and approximately 60% of those with renal stab wounds will have injuries of other intra-abdominal organs which, quite independent of any renal injury, will require surgical exploration and repair.

In terms of blunt injuries, there are two categories of patient in whom a significant renal injury is more likely – those patients who have undergone rapid deceleration and children. Rapid deceleration injuries classically occur in high-speed road traffic accidents and in falls from a height. The kidney in children is said to be more vulnerable to injury because it is proportionately larger, relative to body size, than that of the adult, there is less surrounding perirenal fat and because children have less protective muscle bulk than adults. Indeed, the kidney is the most commonly injured organ in children with blunt abdominal trauma and the most common mechanisms of injury are bicycle and road traffic accidents.

Thus, with this knowledge in mind it is obvious that history-taking plays a crucial role in the assessment of the patient with a renal injury – it indicates the likelihood of a serious renal injury, thus dictating the need for radiological imaging and subsequent management. Examination also provides important clues as to the likelihood of a significant renal injury and therefore of the need for imaging and subsequent exploration.

The key points in history-taking are as follows: is the patient an adult or child, was the injury blunt or penetrating, did it involve a rapid deceleration (any high-speed road traffic accident will obviously have involved sudden deceleration as will a fall from a height), has the patient seen blood in their urine?

In terms of examination the following points must be specifically noted: was any recorded blood pressure <90 mmHg (recorded at any time, either at the scene of the accident or in hospital), is there evidence of a penetrating injury to the flank, lower chest or abdomen? It is worth emphasizing that though blood pressure may be normal when the patient is in the resuscitation room, if at any time prior to this the recorded blood pressure was <90 mmHg, then renal imaging is indicated.

As stated above, patients with renal injuries often have injuries to other organ systems and the general principles of managing the acute trauma victim should therefore be applied while a history and examination are carried out. This will include establishing and maintaining an adequate airway, and gaining intravenous access to allow rapid infusion of fluids and blood as determined by the patient's haemodynamic status.

Investigations

Criteria for radiologic imaging in suspected renal injury. The criteria for radiologic imaging are based on the large trauma experience of McAninch from San Francisco (Mee et al., 1989). Many patients with blunt abdominal injuries have microscopic or dipstick haematuria, but do not have significant renal injuries. These criteria for renal imaging are designed to avoid the need for renal imaging in every patient with abdominal trauma. Renal imaging should be performed in:

(a) penetrating trauma to the flank or abdomen regardless of the extent of haematuria (i.e. whether microscopic or macroscopic);
(b) blunt trauma in adults with gross haematuria;
(c) blunt trauma in adults with microscopic or dipstick haematuria (the presence of bleeding, not the amount, determines the need) and a systolic blood pressure <90 mmHg;
(d) deceleration injury (irrespective of the presence or absence of haematuria);
(e) major intra-abdominal injury with microscopic or dipstick haematuria;
(f) any child with flank or abdominal injury with any degree of haematuria (i.e. whether microscopic or macroscopic).

Thus, adults who sustain blunt trauma, have microscopic haematuria and are normotensive (and have not been hypotensive at any stage) do not need renal imaging, unless the injury was a deceleration one or there is an associated major intra-abdominal injury.

To avoid missing significant renal injuries it is important to appreciate that significant renal injuries may be present in the **absence** of haematuria. This applies to both penetrating abdominal injuries or blunt trauma. This is particularly so with deceleration injuries, which are often associated with renal pedicle (i.e. arterial) injuries which lead to a devascularized kidney – and hence the absence of the source for urinary tract bleeding. Thus, there is no correlation between the degree of haematuria and the extent of renal injury. Clearly haematuria does suggest a possible renal injury, but the key point in abdominal trauma is to consider the possibility of a renal injury based upon the nature of the injury (blunt, penetrating, deceleration etc.).

Any patient with a flank or abdominal penetrating injury who remains haemodynamically unstable despite resuscitation should undergo immediate laparotomy. Surgical exploration should not be delayed to obtain imaging. In such cases on-table single shot intravenous urography can be performed if necessary.

The San Francisco criteria are based on intravenous urography (IVU) (and more latterly CT) as the renal imaging investigation. CT should be used when other abdominal injuries are suspected or when the results of IVU are equivocal. CT has several advantages over IVU. It more accurately stages renal injuries and identifies other intra-abdominal injuries, both factors allowing conservative management to be adopted with greater confidence. While several small series have shown that ultrasound can accurately stage renal injuries and identify those to other intra-abdominal organs, experience in managing renal trauma based on CT or IVU imaging is far greater. It is the extensive experience from the San Francisco General Hospital, based on accurate staging with CT that has allowed a conservative approach to be adopted in most cases of blunt renal injury and many cases of penetrating injury. It is possible that ultrasound may also be able to produce similarly accurate staging – but this has simply not been confirmed in large trauma series.

Imaging allows renal injuries to be identified and staged. Staging is important because it determines subsequent management. Renal injuries are classified according to the American Association for the Surgery of Trauma system (*Table 3.2*).

Criteria for renal imaging in children. The San Francisco recommendations are that all children (aged <16 years) who sustain blunt abdominal trauma and have dipstick haematuria or more than 5 red blood cells per high-power field on microscopy should undergo radiologic imaging, either IVU or CT.

Treatment

The great majority of blunt renal injuries can be managed conservatively, with bed rest and analgesia, and depending on the extent of the initial injury serial CT scans to determine whether there is evidence of an expanding haematoma. A proportion of penetrating renal injuries can also be managed conservatively. In San Francisco approximately 40% of stab wounds and 75% of gunshot wounds require renal exploration. Improved staging, specifically using CT, has allowed a conservative approach to be adopted in many cases.

Absolute indications for renal exploration are persistent hypotension despite resuscitation, an expanding retroperitoneal haematoma (this will usually be identified by serial CT scans) and a pulsatile haematoma (indicating a false aneurysm of a

Table 3.2:
The American Association for the Surgery of Trauma staging system of renal trauma

Grade I	Contusion, subcapsular haematoma; intact renal capsule
Grade II	Minor laceration of the cortex, not involving the medulla or collecting system
Grade III	Major laceration extending through the cortex and medulla, but not involving the collecting system
Grade IV	Major laceration extending through the cortex, medulla and collecting system
Grade V	Shattered kidney (essentially multiple lacerations which split the kidney into multiple fragments) or renal pedicle avulsion or renal artery thrombosis

major renal artery). Relative indications for surgical exploration include extensive urinary extravasation (which indicates a collecting system injury) and arterial thrombosis. Minor degrees of urinary extravasation may be managed expectantly (anticipating spontaneous resolution) or by a ureteric stent which acts to improve urinary drainage.

Ureteric trauma

Because of its retroperitoneal location the ureter is well protected from external trauma. Penetrating trauma is the commonest mechanism of injury. In the UK, where gunshot wounds are rare, most cases of 'penetrating' ureteric injury are related either to pelvic surgery (colorectal or gynaecological) or occur during ureteroscopy. The ureter is vulnerable to injury during pelvic surgery because of its intimate relationship with the broad ligament and uterine artery in women (hence it may be injured during hysterectomy) and the rectosigmoid colon and mesocolon in both sexes.

Blunt ureteric trauma is rare. Deceleration injuries can disrupt the pelviureteric junction, effectively disconnecting the ureter from the kidney.

Presentation

The diagnosis of a ureteric injury will to some extent depend on the clinical context in which the injury occurs. A transected ureter may be obvious at the time of surgery, but if doubt exists about the possibility of a ureteric injury then the ureter can be directly inspected or a retrograde ureterogram can be obtained. Postoperative ureteric injury should be suspected in a patient who develops flank pain, ileus, unexplained pyrexia or drainage of clear fluid from a drain (or healing drain site or abdominal wound) or per vagina (post-hysterectomy). When one suspects drain fluid to be urine a small quantity can be sent for estimation of creatinine level. A creatinine level at or near that of a serum sample confirms that the fluid is lymph; urine will have a much higher creatinine level.

Investigation

Where a ureteric injury is suspected, IVU should be the first line investigation. This will often demonstrate hydronephrosis of the affected kidney, delayed excretion of contrast and absence of contrast in the ureter below the level of the injury. Of course, the entire length of the ureter is not always visualized, even in a normal ureter, and the kidney may not be hydronephrotic if there is free drainage of urine into the abdomen or retroperitoneum from a ureteric transection. Thus, if there is a strong suspicion of a ureteric injury, cystoscopy and retrograde ureterography should be performed. This technique has the advantage that a partial ureteric transection can be stented with a double J ureteric stent at the same time as the procedure, and in some cases this may be all that is necessary to allow the ureteric injury to heal.

Treatment

Primary anastomosis of ureteric injuries that are identified peroperatively is suitable for virtually all injuries other than those involving the distal ureter where a potentially tenuous blood supply can compromise healing. If such an anastomosis is under any degree of tension then it will not heal and a persistent leak of urine will occur. In such cases to bridge a ureteric defect and so avoid tension in the anastomosis, a flap of bladder can be fashioned, swung upwards to bridge the ureteric defect, and then fashioned into a tube into which the ureter is tunnelled. This is called a Boari flap (*Fig. 3.4*). Alternatively, a transverse incision in the wall of the bladder will allow reimplantation of the transected ureter into the bladder, any discrepancy in ureteric length being overcome by closing the bladder incision longitudinally, so effectively lengthening the bladder in a vertical direction (*Fig. 3.5*). The bladder is held in its new location by several 'hitch' sutures, which hold the bladder onto the psoas minor tendon, hence the technique is called the 'psoas hitch'. If the length of injured ureter is very large, and reimplantation into the bladder is not feasible, then the affected ureter may be swung across to the opposite ureter (behind the mesentery of the bowel) and anastomosed to this ureter. This is called a transureteroureterostomy (or TUU).

Where the diagnosis of a ureteric injury is made post-operatively an attempt at insertion of a ureteric 'double J' stent at the time of retrograde

Fig. 3.4:
Diagram demonstrating the principle of the Boari flap for managing lower ureteric injuries.

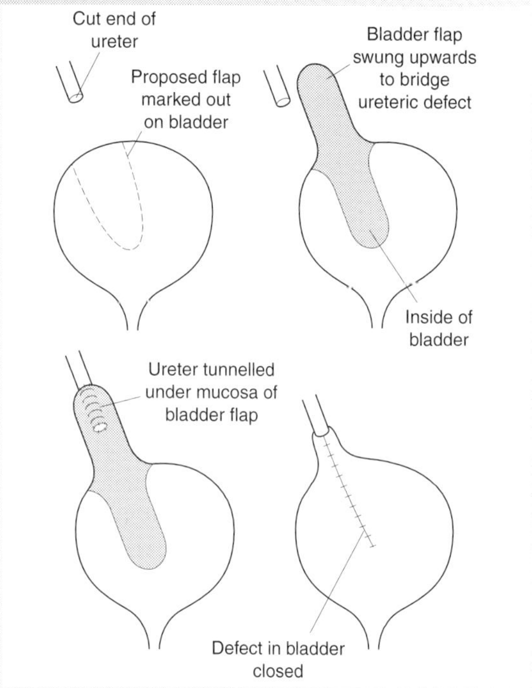

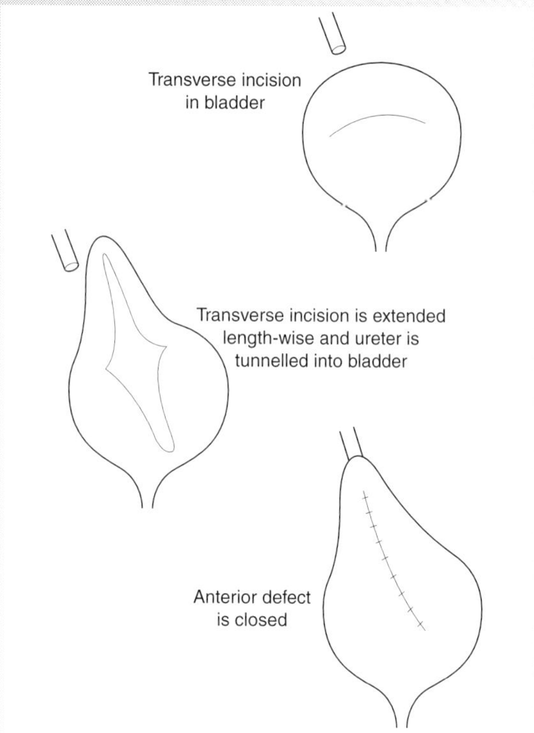

ureterography can be made. If a guidewire can be passed across the area of injury, so allowing access to the non-injured ureter above, then it is usually possible to pass a stent. If there is a demonstrable collection of urine around the site of ureteric injury, a percutaneous drain can be placed with radiological screening. If a double J stent cannot be passed then open surgical repair by one of the techniques described above should be the next step.

Bladder trauma

The mechanisms of bladder injury are specific. As with renal injures, a carefully taken history should alert you to the possibility that a bladder injury might have occurred.

Presentation

The bladder may be injured at the time of endoscopic bladder surgery (transurethral resection of

Fig. 3.5:
Diagram demonstrating the principle of the psoas hitch procedure which allows the bladder to be extended upwards, so bridging a lower ureteric defect.

bladder tumour is the classic culprit) or pelvic surgery, particularly caesarian section. Such injuries are usually obvious at the time of the procedure. Traumatic bladder injuries occur as a result of either a blow to the lower abdomen, particularly when the bladder is full, or in association with pelvic fracture, where a sharp bone edge from the fractured pelvis can directly damage the bladder. Penetrating (externally penetrating) bladder injuries are unusual in the UK, but obviously a penetrating wound in the lower abdomen should alert you to the possibility that the bladder may have been injured. Spontaneous rupture of the bladder can occur in patients who have undergone previous bladder augmentation (where a segment of detubularized bowel is stitched onto the dome of the bladder in order to increase its capacity).

The patient with a bladder injury will usually complain of lower abdominal or suprapubic pain (though patients with neurological disorders such as spina bifida or spinal cord injuries – some of whom may have had a bladder augmentation – may not do so and this can lead to a delay in diagnosis). The other symptoms of a bladder injury include difficulty or inability to void (a bladder which is emptying into the peritoneal cavity obviously may not empty per urethra) and haematuria. Examination may reveal lower abdominal tenderness and an ileus with abdominal distension and absent bowel sounds.

Investigation

Retrograde cystography is the most accurate method of diagnosing a bladder injury. This involves the passage of a urethral catheter, instillation of contrast into the bladder and X-ray screening to identify a leak. Generally speaking at least 400 ml of contrast should be instilled into the bladder. A small perforation can be plugged by small-bowel or omentum, and this may not be apparent if lower volumes of contrast, resulting in inadequate bladder distension, are used. Once this has been done all of the contrast should be drained from the bladder and a post-drainage film taken. Sometimes a small leak of contrast may be obscured by the presence of dense contrast in a full bladder and may only be apparent when the contrast has been drained from the bladder.

Treatment

Retrograde cystography allows classification of bladder injuries into those that are extraperitoneal and those that are intraperitoneal; the former obviously being contained within the pelvis with no leak of urine into the peritoneal cavity. This is a useful classification system because it determines subsequent treatment. Extraperitoneal perforations can, generally speaking, be managed by a period of catheter drainage (with antibiotic cover throughout this period) and the majority will heal within 10 to 14 days (some take a little longer). Confirmation of healing can be obtained by a repeat cystogram. Intraperitoneal bladder perforations, on the other hand, should be managed by open surgical repair, again with post-operative bladder catheter drainage.

One word of warning: bladder injuries may coexist with urethral injuries, particularly when there is a pelvic fracture. When blood is present at the meatus, or if it is absent but a catheter will not pass into the bladder, a retrograde urethrogram should be performed to exclude a urethral injury. Though the presence of visible blood at the urethral meatus is often due to a urethral injury in isolation, it must be remembered that it could also be coming from either a bladder or renal injury. As stated above (**Renal trauma**) any trauma patient with macroscopic haematuria should undergo renal imaging and in the context of urethral bleeding, bladder imaging should also be done. Of course, if a urethral catheter cannot be passed into the bladder because of a urethral disruption, then a retrograde cystogram cannot be done. In such a situation how can one adequately visualize the bladder? A suprapubic catheter should be placed either percutaneously, or (more commonly) by formal open cystostomy, through a short transverse lower abdominal incision with direct visualization and catheterization of the bladder. If a percutaneous suprapubic catheter has been placed then a cystogram can be obtained via this catheter. If an open cystostomy is done then the inside of the bladder can be directly inspected at the time of the procedure.

Urethral trauma

Urethral injuries may involve the anterior urethra or posterior urethra. The anterior urethra extends from the external urethral meatus to the distal end of the membranous urethra (wherein lies the external urethral sphincter). The posterior urethra includes the membranous urethra (and therefore the external sphincter) and the prostatic urethra.

The mechanism of injury to the anterior urethra is very different from that in injuries of the posterior urethra. The former are caused by instrumentation (cystoscopy, catheterization, including inflating a catheter balloon in the urethra or removal of a catheter with the balloon inflated) or fall astride injuries (little boys – or men – forcefully hitting the cross bar of their bicycles or receiving a blow to the perineum). This crushes the bulbar urethra against the inferior pubis. More rarely the anterior urethra may be torn when the erect penis is forcibly bent, which literally fractures the corpora cavernosa and sometimes the corpus spongiosum, within which the anterior urethra runs. Posterior urethral injuries on the other hand are usually due to pelvic fractures, which usually require massive force. Posterior urethral injuries are therefore often associated with damage to major pelvic blood vessels, resulting in life-threatening blood loss. The management of anterior and posterior urethral injuries is therefore very different.

Presentation of anterior urethral injuries

Once again, history-taking is very important in reaching a correct diagnosis. A history of a fall astride injury or other blow to the perineum should arouse your suspicion that there may be an anterior urethral injury. The patient may be unable to void. Examination may reveal blood at the external meatus or bruising of the penis, perineum or lower abdomen, the exact distribution being determined by which layer of penile fascia has been disrupted. Buck's fascia is a tube of connective tissue surrounding the corpora cavernosa and corpus spongiosum. Proximally it fuses with the tunica albuginea of the corpora (the tunica albuginea is the thick, cylindrical tube of connective tissue that encases each corpus) and this fusion of Buck's fascia with the corpora prevents further spread of any extravasated blood. Thus, an anterior urethral injury which does not rupture Buck's fascia will result in penile bruising that is confined to the shaft of the penis. If Buck's fascia is ruptured, the bruising is then confined by the next (more superficial) layer of connective tissue, Colles fascia. Colles fascia fuses posteriorly with the perineal body and extends a little way down each thigh. Bleeding beneath this layer of fascia will thus create bruising of a characteristic pattern in the perineum, the so-called butterfly bruising of anterior urethral rupture (*Fig. 3.6*). Colles fascia is renamed Scarpa's fascia as it sweeps upwards into the abdomen. Superiorly it is attached to the clavicles, so if Buck's fascia is ruptured allowing blood to extravasate beneath Colles fascia and if the bleeding from an anterior urethral injury is extensive enough, bruising may extend all the way to the clavicles.

Fig. 3.6:
Butterfly bruising of the perineum in anterior urethral rupture.

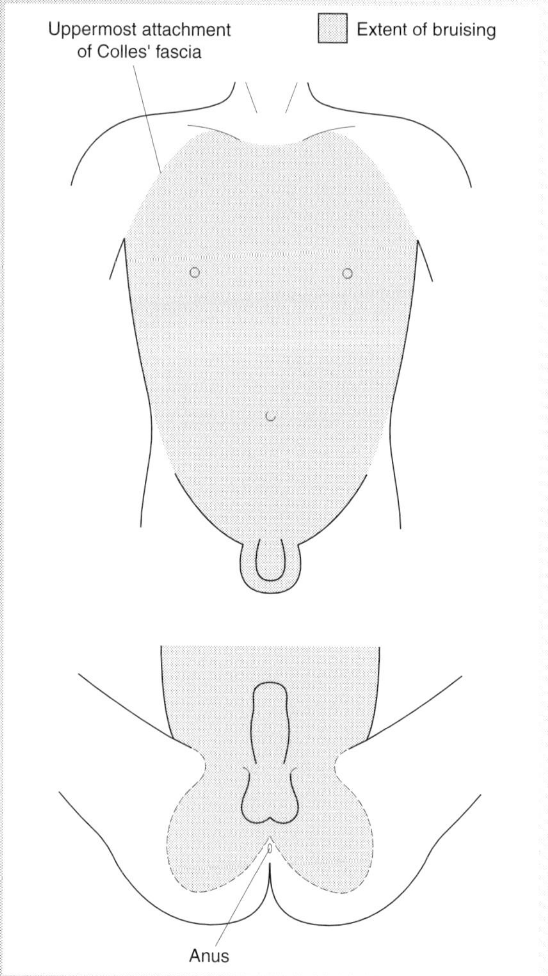

Investigation

Retrograde urethrography is used to identify the presence of a urethral injury (*Fig. 3.7*). A small (e.g. 12 Ch) catheter is inserted with its tip just inside the urethral meatus and the balloon inflated to prevent it from falling out (alternatively a penile

Fig. 3.7:
A normal retrograde urethrogram. Note that there is a narrowing (normal) of the urethra as it passes through the urogenital diaphragm (the urogenital membrane). This marks the level of the membranous urethra, and is the site of the external urethral sphincter.

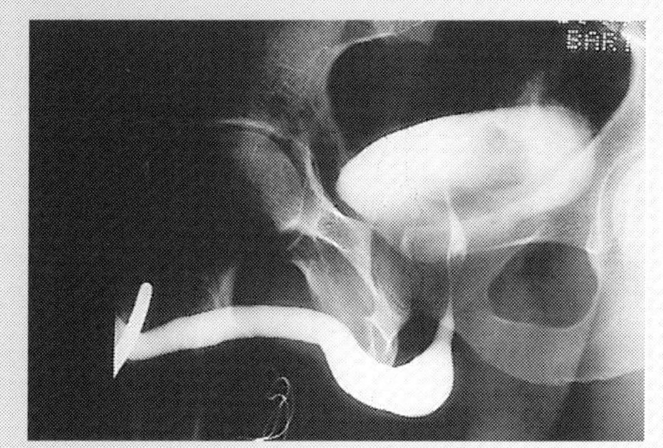

clamp can be applied to the end of the penis to stop contrast from flowing out of the penis on injection). Water soluble contrast is injected and screening performed during the injection. Extravasation of contrast confirms a urethral injury. A patient who has sustained a fall astride injury, and who has blood at the external meatus, but no extravasation is said to have an anterior urethral contusion.

The acute treatment of anterior urethral injuries

Anterior urethral contusions can be managed by advancing a small-bore silicone catheter (12 Ch) into the bladder and this is left on free drainage for 10 to 14 days. Broad-spectrum antibiotics are prescribed. Patients with extravasation (indicating incomplete or complete anterior urethral disruption) should be managed by suprapubic catheterization – so diverting urine away from the site of injury while the urethra heals. Urethral catheterization can convert an incomplete disruption to a complete one, and may introduce infection into the haematoma. The segment of intact urethral mucosa will allow re-epithelialization of the urethra and while some patients may subsequently develop a stricture, many of these are mild and of no functional significance. Voiding urethrography (introduction of contrast into the bladder, clamping of the suprapubic tube, followed by the patient passing urine) 3 to 4 weeks later will determine whether the urethra has healed, at which time the suprapubic catheter can be removed.

In cases of penetrating anterior urethral injury or those associated with penile fracture, primary repair of the urethra should be performed over a urethral catheter.

Presentation and investigation of posterior urethral injuries

As stated above, posterior urethral injuries usually occur as a consequence of pelvic fracture (*Fig. 3.8a, 3.8b*), and are thus often associated with life-threatening pelvic bleeding (from torn pelvic veins) and other injuries, both abdominal and chest as well as head injuries and other fractures. Bladder and renal injuries may coexist with the posterior urethral disruption. Catheterization is important to allow monitoring of urine output in patients who are likely to be haemodynamically unstable, and also to establish urinary drainage, so preventing leakage of urine into the pelvis.

The haemodynamically unstable patient. Whether a retrograde urethrogram is obtained in the emergency room will depend on the need for urgent surgery for treatment of associated injuries. The patient may have coexistent intra-abdominal bleeding necessitating urgent laparotomy – obviously there may not be time to obtain a retrograde urethrogram in such a case. In this instance a gentle attempt should be made to catheterize the bladder in the operating theatre, and any resistance to catheterization will indicate the need for placement of a suprapubic catheter at the time of laparotomy.

Treatment of posterior urethral injuries

Placement of a suprapubic catheter under direct vision at the time of laparotomy is usually safer than percutaneous catheterization (see below), as long as the pelvic haematoma is not disturbed, and it affords the possibility of inspecting the inside of the bladder for injuries, which should be repaired at that time.

Fig. 3.8:
(a) A pelvic fracture resulting from the patient being run-over by a car. (b) Retrograde urethrogram from the same patient showing a urethral disruption. The anterior urethra has been disconnected from the posterior urethra (the bladder and attached prostate having risen upwards). Contrast cannot pass beyond the bulbar urethra. Contrast has also been injected into the bladder via a suprapubic catheter.

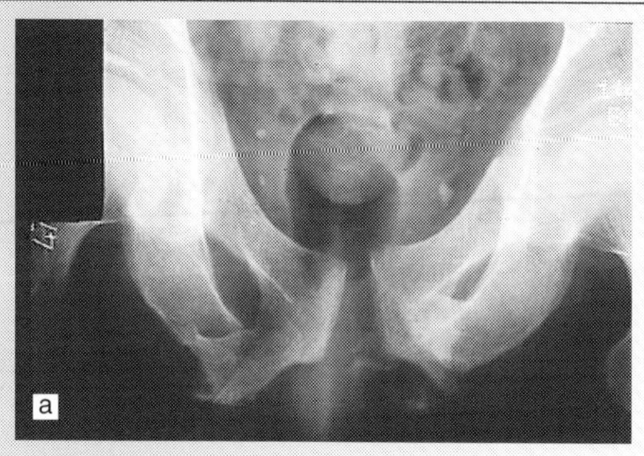

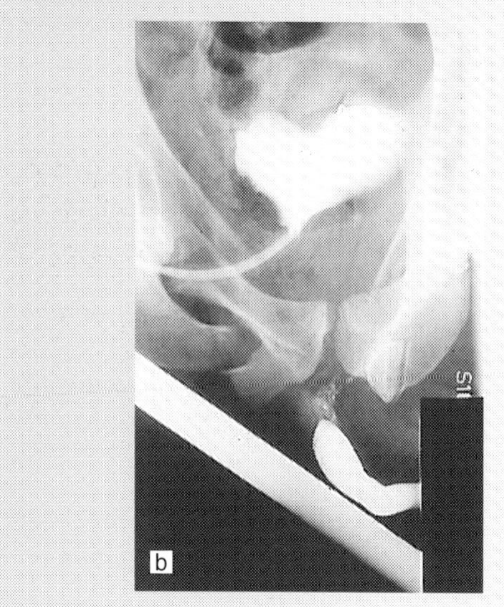

The haemodynamically stable patient. In the stable patient with a pelvic fracture in whom urgent laparotomy is **not** required and where there is **no** blood at the external meatus, a gentle attempt at catheterization should be made. If the catheter passes easily into the bladder and clear urine with no haematuria is obtained then a bladder injury is unlikely and a formal cystogram is not necessary, though it can certainly be comforting if a cystogram is obtained and it is normal. Any resistance to passage of the catheter indicates the need for retrograde urethrography. If this demonstrates a posterior urethral rupture, whether partial or complete, then a suprapubic catheter should be placed. Again, formal open cystostomy (direct exposure of the bladder via a suprapubic incision) is better than percutaneous suprapubic catheterization because (1) it allows accurate placement of the catheter in the bladder – in the presence of a pelvic fracture it is all too easy to catheterize the pelvis haematoma or the peritoneal cavity, with the potential for bowel perforation. Perforating bowel is a serious complication in any situation, but contamination of a pelvic haematoma with bowel organisms could lead to life-threatening sepsis; (2) it allows associated bladder injuries to be identified and repaired. A catheter may not necessarily provide adequate urinary diversion if there is an associated bladder injury. Failure to repair such injuries may lead to extravasation of urine, which again may lead to the potentially disastrous consequence of infection of the pelvic haematoma.

Blood at the external urethral meatus is an indication for retrograde urethrography. No attempt at urethral catheterization should be made. If the urethra is normal, the catheter may be advanced into the bladder and a cystogram should be done to determine whether a bladder injury is present. If the posterior urethra is disrupted, a suprapubic catheter is inserted and a delayed anastomotic urethroplasty performed to restore continuity 3 months later. Most patients with a pelvic fracture will undergo an abdominal as well as pelvic CT scan, so it is unlikely that significant renal injuries will be missed, but it is worth repeating that any trauma patient with macroscopic haematuria (even if this is a small amount at the external urethral meatus) should have imaging of the kidneys (IVU or better still a CT scan).

Testicular trauma

This is usually caused by blunt trauma. A significant force is required to disrupt the tough tunica albuginea of the testis. The contained seminiferous tubules extrude through a tear in the tunica and accompanying haemorrhage results in formation of a scrotal haematoma.

Presentation and investigation

Sporting injuries are the most common cause of testicular trauma, but injury may also occur from assaults or motor vehicle accidents. Not surprisingly the patient will be in considerable pain and there may be a tense scrotal swelling. Ultrasound is very useful in staging the degree of testicular injury and thus in determining subsequent management. On ultrasound the parenchyma of the normal testis (the substance of the testis contained within the tunica albuginea) is characterized by a uniform pattern of medium-intensity echoes. In testicular rupture (rupture of the tunica albuginea), focal areas of hypogenicity appear in the parenchyma. A tear may be seen in the tunica, but absence of a tear does not exclude a rupture. A haematoma surrounding the testis may be seen.

Focal areas of parenchymal hypogenicity on ultrasound and particularly haematomas surrounding the testis are often associated with testicular rupture. A testicular rupture is usually taken as an indication for exploration and repair of the torn tunica albuginea because series of testicular trauma have shown that patients managed by exploration have a shorter hospital stay, a reduced orchidectomy rate and earlier return to normal activities. It is possible that evacuation of a haematoma may relieve pressure on the testis and so reduce the likelihood of subsequent ischaemic damage.

Penile fracture

This relatively unusual condition is caused by a tear of the corpora cavernosa. It is an injury that only occurs to the erect penis, since the corpora must be rigid. The injury usually occurs during rigorous intercourse by forcibly bending the erection against the pubic arch.

Presentation

The patient may report a sudden loud, cracking noise as the penis fractures and will notice sudden and rapid detumescence (i.e. loss of rigidity) and pain. This is accompanied by marked swelling and bruising of the penis. The end result after some hours is the so-called 'aubergine' deformity (*Fig. 3.9*). It is important to ask the patient if they have been able to void urine following the injury, and if so whether they noticed blood in their urine. Fracture of the corpus spongiosum, through which the urethra passes, will cause a urethral tear (which may be partial or complete) and this occurs in 10–20% of cases of penile fracture. The meatus should be examined for the presence of blood, but the absence of blood at the meatus does not exclude a urethral injury and the urine should also be dipsticked, any degree of haematuria being an indication for retrograde urethrography.

Investigation

The diagnosis is essentially a clinical one, based on a characteristic history and physical appearance. Further examination may reveal a palpable deformity in the shaft of the penis, but swelling and tenderness are usually too marked to allow this to be identified. Ultrasound scanning has been

Fig. 3.9:
A fractured penis. The characteristic swelling and bruising gives the appearance of an aubergine!

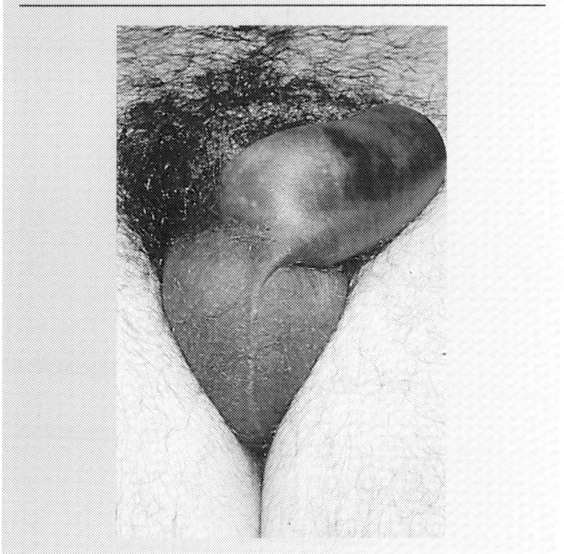

used to demonstrate the site of fracture, and enthusiasts have even reported the use of MRI to diagnose this condition! Because associated urethral injuries are relatively common and may not always be manifest by the presence of meatal blood, one should have a low threshold for performing a retrograde urethrogram. This is a simple and reliable test.

Treatment

Since there are no randomized studies comparing conservative against surgical treatment, penile fracture may be managed either way. Proponents of conservative treatment state that the condition will eventually resolve spontaneously and that any subsequent deformity of the erect penis can be corrected at a later date if the patient so wishes. Proponents of immediate surgical exploration and repair of the tear state that the penile swelling resolves more rapidly with such an approach and that penile deformity is less likely to occur. A circumcision is usually undertaken after de-gloving the penis.

The presence of an associated incomplete urethral tear can be managed in several ways. An attempt at urethral catheterization can be made, the catheter serving both to divert urine from the tear (so there is no extravasation of urine) and also as a splint around which the urethra may heal. Alternatively, the urine may be diverted via a suprapubic catheter (see **Anterior urethral injuries** above). A third option is primary surgical repair. There are advocates of all these approaches, and again there are no hard and fast rules. A complete urethral tear should be repaired surgically at the time of presentation.

Penile amputation

Though this is rare problem, it is clearly a very dramatic presentation and is mentioned because if the case is managed appropriately, the penis may be reimplanted and remain viable. Given the high blood flow to the penis there may obviously be considerable blood loss in cases of penile amputation and the patient is likely to need resuscitation before an attempt at reimplantation can be made. From the point of view of early management it is important to be aware that successful reimplantation of the penis (at least in terms of viability if not erectile function) may be achieved even if the penis has been normothermic (i.e. not stored under hypothermic conditions) for many hours. The penis has been successfully reimplanted after 16 hours of 'warm' ischaemia. Storing the amputated penis under hypothermic conditions will clearly prolong its survival and increase the likelihood of graft take.

If you are confronted with a patient with an amputated penis, wash it gently in saline and then wrap it in a saline-soaked gauze and place in a clean plastic bag which should be sealed. This is then placed in a second bag (or other container), which is full of ice-slush (ice and water) – 'a bag in a bag'. Transport this with the patient to hospital.

Key points

Renal trauma

- Degree of haematuria correlates poorly with extent of renal injury.
- Rapid deceleration injuries can be associated with significant renal injuries in the absence of even microscopic haematuria.
- CT scanning provides the most accurate method of identifying and staging renal injuries and the trend is away from IVU. Ultrasound is not commonly used for renal imaging in the trauma setting.
- Virtually all blunt renal injuries can be managed conservatively.
- Most penetrating injuries will require exploration to stop continued bleeding and treat associated injuries.

Urethral trauma

- Considerable force is required to injure the posterior urethra (as opposed to the anterior urethra) and is usually associated with a major pelvic fracture, severe pelvic bleeding and associated chest and abdominal injuries.
- The presence of blood at the external urethral meatus often indicates the presence of a urethral injury.
- Attempted catheterization should be performed by an experienced doctor and any resistance to catheterization is an indication (in the stable patient) for retrograde urethrography.

Urinary retention

- You cannot diagnose urinary retention or the type of retention without recording the volume of urine obtained on catheterization of the bladder.

Ureteric colic

- 50% of cases of suspected 'ureteric colic' do not have ureteric stones.

Cases

1. A 28-year-old man is brought into casualty having crashed his motorbike at 60 mph. His systolic blood pressure at the scene was 80 mmHg, but is now 110 mmHg after a litre of a plasma expander has been infused. He is complaining of left loin pain. He has dipstick haematuria on urine testing.
   (a) Does he require renal imaging?
   (b) What imaging test would you recommend?
   (c) His scan shows a large retroperitoneal haematoma, with a major laceration extending through the cortex and medulla of his left kidney, but not involving the collecting system. What should subsequent management of these findings be?

2. A 24-year-old male has been run-over by a lorry and is brought into casualty unconscious. His systolic blood pressure is 120 mmHg. His plain abdominal X-ray is shown in *Figure 3.8a*. You are asked to pass a urethral catheter to allow measurement of his urine output.
   (a) What examination should you perform prior to passing a catheter?
   (b) There is no blood at his meatus and you pass the catheter, but it stops approximately 15 cm down his urethra and will go no further. What should you do next?
   (c) The retrograde urethrogram shows extravasation of contrast into his perineum. No contrast flows into his bladder. What is the diagnosis? How should a catheter be placed in his bladder?

3. A 70-year-old man presents with painful inability to void and reports bedwetting every night for the last 6 weeks. On urethral catheterization 2.5 l of urine is drained. His serum creatinine is 400 mmol l^{-1} and 2 days later this has fallen to 150 mmol l^{-1}.
   (a) What is the diagnosis?
   (b) What measurements should be performed on a regular basis in the first few days of his admission?

Answers

1. (a) The nature of his accident (high-velocity road traffic acccident, likely to have involved rapid deceleration) is, in itself, an indication for renal imaging as is the fact that he was hypotensive at some stage post-injury and has a degree of haematuria.
   (b) CT scanning of his abdomen will provide the most accurate way of staging a suspected renal injury and will also allow accurate staging of an associated splenic injury, which should be excluded given his left loin pain.
   (c) As long as he remains haemodynamically stable this injury can be managed expectantly with bed rest and analgesia. Cross-matched blood should be kept available in case he suddenly drops his blood pressure – an indication of possible on-going bleeding.

2. (a) Look at his meatus for evidence of blood. If this is present you must obtain a retrograde urethrogram prior to attempting to pass the catheter (assuming he is haemodynamically stable allowing you time to obtain this investigation). Digital rectal examination in such a case should also be done, principally to exclude an associated rectal injury, which you should suspect if there is blood when you withdraw your finger.
   (b) This is another indication for a retrograde urethrogram.
   (c) His prostate has been disconnected (partially or completely) from his anterior urethra. Measurement of urine output in this patient is crucial so a catheter must be passed into his bladder. Furthermore, failure to do so could result in extravasation of urine into his pelvic haematoma. A catheter should be passed by formal open suprapubic cystostomy in the operating theatre, keeping well away from his pelvic haematoma (so as not to cause further bleeding or introduce infection).

3. (a) He has high pressure chronic retention of urine. The fall in creatinine following relief of his bladder outlet obstruction suggests high intra-renal pressures have developed as a consequence of his retention.
   (b) Urine output should be measured on an hourly basis and lying and standing blood pressure every few hours. The latter measurements will indicate whether he is becoming intravascularly volume depleted, and is used as an indication for fluid replacement with Normal saline. Daily measurement of serum creatinine will allow you to monitor the recovery in his renal function.

References

Dahm P., Roland F.H., Vaslef S.N. et al. Outcome analysis in patients with primary necrotizing fasciitis of the male genitalia. *Urology* 2000; **56**: 31–36.

Mee S.L., McAninch J.W., Robinson A.L. et al. Radiographic assessment of renal trauma: a 10 year prospective study of patient selection. *J Urol* 1989; **141**: 1095.

Reynard J.M., Shearer R.J. Failure to void after TURP and mode of presentation. *Urology* 1999; **53**: 336–339.

CHAPTER 4

Bladder outlet obstruction

Causes of bladder outlet obstruction (BOO)

This is very much dependent on the age of the patient. In male neonates with BOO the cause is likely to be congenital urethral valves or obstructing embryological remnants. In younger men urethral strictures or functional bladder neck obstruction are common causes of obstruction (though obstruction is unusual in young men). Bladder neck dyssynergia and, more rarely, neurological causes such as detrusor sphincter dyssynergia (Chapter 6) and static distal sphincter obstruction can also cause BOO in younger men. In older males benign prostatic obstruction (BPO) due to benign prostatic enlargement (BPE) is the commonest cause of BOO – up to 70% of men in their seventh decade of life. Other causes of BOO in the elderly male include obstruction from prostate cancer, urethral stricture, or urethral foreign bodies (which include urethral stones).

In women obstruction may be due to urethral strictures, pelvic masses (which can occlude the urethra) such as ovarian or fibroid uterine masses, previous anti-incontinence surgery, prolapse (cystocele, rectocele, uterine), primary bladder neck obstruction, and urethral diverticulum or, in some cases may be due to urethral dysfunction (a functional obstruction, with no demonstrable anatomical abnormality occurring in the neurologically normal). Some women with LUTS (lower urinary tract symptoms) or urinary retention have been found to have abnormal EMG activity in the urethral sphincter, and it is believed that this is associated with inadequate relaxation of the urethral sphincter, leading to obstruction to the flow of urine and ultimately retention (Fowler and Kirby, 1986).

Modes of presentation of BOO

There are two main ways in which BOO may present – acute retention of urine or LUTS. Urinary retention in males is covered in Chapter 3. An uncommon presentation of BOO is with a bladder stone, which may itself cause haematuria, bladder pain or both.

While LUTS may certainly be caused by BOO, in recent years we have come to appreciate that men presenting with urinary symptoms may not have obstruction. In traditional urological teaching, benign prostatic hyperplasia (BPH) causes benign prostatic enlargement (BPE), which by compressing the urethra causes bladder outlet obstruction (BOO). This in turn leads to a complex of symptoms, classically called 'prostatism' and, if a critical degree of BOO ensues urinary retention may occur. This concept has been thrown into question by the observation that age-matched elderly men and women have equivalent 'BPH' symptom scores (despite the obvious absence of a prostate in women!) and by a wealth of data which has failed to find any close correlation between urinary symptoms, prostatic enlargement and BOO. We therefore nowadays talk about LUTS rather than prostatism (Abrams, 1994), since the term prostatism implies a pathophysiological significance which simply does not exist ('prostatism' implies the symptoms are due to the prostate). It is important to appreciate that LUTS have no real diagnostic value – they simply tell you that something is wrong, but not precisely what is wrong. The presence of LUTS cannot therefore, in themselves, be used to diagnose BOO.

LUTS are subdivided into so-called storage symptoms (frequency, urgency and nocturia), since they occur at a time when the bladder should be storing urine, and voiding symptoms (hesitancy, poor urinary flow, intermittent flow and terminal dribbling) which occur during the process of voiding. A number of symptom scores have been developed to quantify symptoms and measure the 'bothersomeness' of those symptoms. The most well known is the AUA (American Urological Association) score (it is also known as the International Prostate Symptom Score or IPSS). More recently the International Continence Society has developed a validated symptom questionnaire, one for men and another for women, which provides a very comprehensive record of a patient's symptoms. The AUA symptom score asks the patient to rate the severity of 7 symptoms – poor flow, intermittency, straining, incomplete bladder emptying, frequency, nocturia and urgency. Each symptom is rated from 0 to 5, depending on whether the symptom is absent or occurs less than 20% of the time, less than half the time, half the time, more than half the time or almost always. The highest possible total score is 35. The AUA symptom score also asks the patient to 'score' the overall bother that their symptoms cause them by asking 'If you were to spend the rest of your life with your urinary condition just the way it is now, how would you feel about that?'. The responses (and appropriate scores) are delighted (0), pleased (1), mostly satisfied (2), mixed – satisfied and dissatisfied (3), mostly dissatisfied (4), unhappy (5) and terrible (6).

When the AUA symptom score was first developed it was thought that it would be able to diagnose BPH or BOO, but as discussed above, individual symptoms or summations of symptoms (into scores) are not able to discriminate patients with BOO from those without. Nonetheless, they do allow a record of a patient's symptoms to be made, which can be used to document the effect of various treatments.

Having said that, symptoms have no real diagnostic power; some symptoms are suggestive of underlying pathology. Macroscopic haematuria, particularly in those aged over 50 is associated with a urological malignancy (bladder or kidney) in a substantial proportion of patients and the symptom of bedwetting is very suggestive of high-pressure chronic retention. One should also be suspicious of the patient with marked urgency or bladder pain (i.e. suprapubic pain) for this may indicate the presence of an underlying bladder cancer, particularly carcinoma in situ (malignant cystitis). Many urologists arrange for such patients to have a cystoscopy, to allow direct visualization of the bladder.

Examination of the patient presenting with LUTS should include suprapubic palpation and percussion for the presence of an enlarged bladder, a digital rectal examination (DRE) to assess whether the prostate has a benign or malignant consistency and a focused neurological examination. In cases where a neurological basis for the symptoms is suspected, this should include eliciting the bulbocavernosus reflex (squeezing the glans penis gently, but firmly while performing a DRE and eliciting contraction of the anus – a test of the integrity of the sacral cord and its afferent and efferent connections to the bladder), eliciting the ankle reflex and testing sensation in the feet and perianal region.

Assessment of prostate size by digital rectal examination is inaccurate, though it can give a rough indication of prostatic size. If the prostate appears to be large on DRE, a transrectal ultrasound (TRUS) provides a very accurate measurement of size. While the correlation between prostate size and BOO is poor, pre-operative assessment of prostatic size indicates the particular operative approach to prostatectomy. Small prostates can be managed by transurethral prostatectomy (TURP); very large prostates are best removed by open prostatectomy.

Pathophysiology of BPO

There are believed to be two components to prostatic obstruction – obstruction due to increased tone of prostatic smooth muscle (which is innervated by sympathetic nerves – this is the so-called dynamic component) and that due to the bulk effect of the enlarged prostate (the so-called static component). One component may be more important than another in a particular individual, and this may be part of the explanation why prostate size correlates relatively poorly with degree of obstruction as measured by pressure–flow studies.

Investigation of a patient with suspected BOO

As stated above, LUTS suggest that the patient has some bladder or urethral pathology, but not *which* pathology. Further investigations are required to establish whether the patient's symptoms are caused by underlying BOO.

Uroflowmetry records maximum flow rate (Q_{max} – measured in $ml\,s^{-1}$) against time. Nowadays, computerized flowmeters are available, which provide a print-out of Q_{max} against time, and give additional information such as voided volume (see *Figs. 2.9–2.11*). The test is non-invasive and simple. There is a statistical relationship between flow rate and presence of BOO. Thus, in one study of almost 1300 men with LUTS (Reynard et al., 1998) those with BOO had a Q_{max} of $9.7\,ml\,s^{-1}$ compared with $12.6\,ml\,s^{-1}$ in those without BOO. However, some men with BOO had high flows, and other men with no BOO had low flows. Using a cut-off value of Q_{max} of $<10\,ml\,s^{-1}$ as indicating the presence of BOO gave a specificity for diagnosing BOO of 70%, a sensitivity of 47% and a positive predictive value of 70%. Thus, uroflowmetry alone (specifically Q_{max}) cannot be used with certainty to diagnose BOO. This is because a low flow can be due to an underactive detrusor, rather than to the presence of BOO (i.e. there may be no restriction to flow in the urethra, but the pressure head that the bladder is able to produce is low – hence Q_{max} will be low). More complex **urodynamic investigation**, where pressure as well as flow is measured (pressure–flow studies) is required to determine whether the patient has obstruction or not.

Residual urine volume can be measured by ultrasonography. This provides an accurate measurement of residual volume. As with uroflowmetry the correlation between residual urine volume and presence of BOO is poor – so the presence of residual urine does not imply the presence of BOO.

Pressure–flow studies provide information about bladder pressure at the peak value for Q_{max} and there are a variety of methods (equations and nomograms), which relate pressure to flow and allow one to diagnose the presence or absence of BOO. One such nomogram is known as the ICS provisional nomogram (*Fig. 4.1*) and it is a derivative of the older (and more well known) Abrams–Griffiths nomogram (Griffiths et al., 1997). Values for pressure and flow are determined from the pressure–flow study, and a diagnosis of BOO can thus be made. **Pressure–flow studies are the gold-standard method (indeed the only method) for diagnosing BOO.**

Fig. 4.1:
The ICS provisional nomogram.

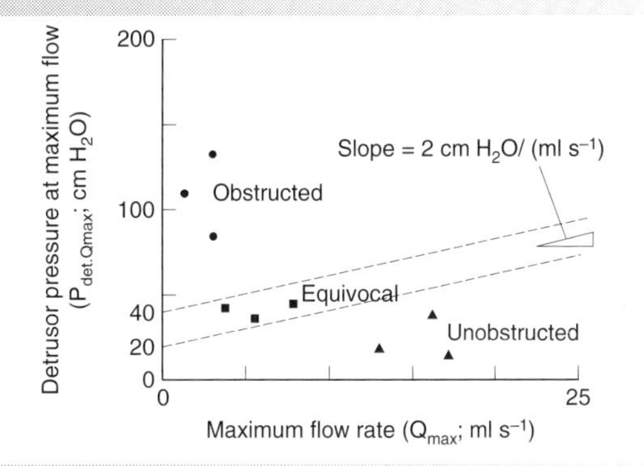

Redrawn by permission of Wiley-Liss Inc., a subsidiary of John Wiley & Sons Inc. from Standardisation of terminology of lower urinary tract function: pressure–flow studies of voiding, urethral resistance and urethral obstruction, Griffiths D. *et al.*, *Neurourol Urodyn*, © 1997 Wiley-Liss Inc.

However, whether one proceeds to pressure–flow studies in the 'average' elderly patient presenting with LUTS, whom you suspect has benign prostatic obstruction, depends to some degree on your philosophy about what you are trying to treat. Most people would agree that we should treat symptoms. Some believe that as long as the symptoms improve, it doesn't matter whether the patient has obstruction or not, and therefore why bother attempting to diagnose BOO if the diagnosis is not going to influence response to treatment? Similarly, some argue that measurement of post-void residual urine volume and Q_{max} are of no value in predicting outcome of treatment – and therefore why bother measuring these urodynamic variables? Thus, in the United States the Agency for Health Care Policy and Research (McConnell et al., 1994) has issued 'Clinical Practice Guidelines' for management of men with LUTS that concluded 'establishing a precise diagnosis is of minimal value if the information does not lead to a difference in clinical outcome'. The whole area of diagnosis of LUTS has been the source of much debate over the last few years.

In the Veterans Affairs trial of TURP versus watchful waiting, men with a PVR of 100 ml or less had no significant difference in symptom reduction after TURP compared to those with a PVR 101–350 ml (Bruskewitz et al., 1997) and Q_{max} could not predict who would have a successful outcome and who would not. While pressure–flow studies can certainly determine whether a patient has BOO, again their prognostic value with respect to the outcome of prostatectomy is questionable. In men selected for prostatectomy on the basis of symptoms and a Q_{max} <15 ml s^{-1}, Neal et al. (1989) reported a poor outcome in 21% of those with BOO compared with 36% in those without BOO. However, most of those without obstruction did well and pressure–flow studies were unable to predict the likelihood of a poor outcome in individual cases. Essentially, while men with BOO confirmed on pressure–flow studies statistically have a greater chance of improvement in their LUTS post-TURP, most patients with LUTS who have not undergone formal pressure–flow studies (and proceed to TURP solely on the basis of their LUTS) also have a good symptomatic outcome. The proponents of pressure–flow studies say that the cost-savings from performing pressure–flow studies and not operating on men with no evidence of BOO, offset the costs of the pressure–flow studies. However, as 60% of men without BOO report improvement in their LUTS after TURP, it is difficult to deny them a potentially beneficial treatment, simply because they do not fit into a certain diagnostic category.

Most patients presenting with LUTS are seeking a treatment that will improve their symptoms, and may not be particularly interested in establishing for certain that these symptoms are due to BOO. In the UK, pressure–flow studies are not part of the routine diagnostic evaluation of elderly men with LUTS who are thought to have BPO. Investigation of a patient with suspected BOO therefore usually centres around the nature of his symptoms (which can be assessed by direct questioning or by symptom score) and this is usually supplemented by measurement of flow rate (though as mentioned above the evidence for measurement of Q_{max} being of prognostic value is not good). A definite diagnosis of BOO is therefore not usually obtained and the patient is treated in the absence of a definite urodynamic diagnosis. We are therefore really discussing investigation of the patient with suspected BOO.

There are certainly patients who are not 'average' and in whom pressure–flow studies can provide useful diagnostic information, particularly when combined with simultaneous X-ray screening of the bladder neck and urethra during voiding. These include younger patients with LUTS in whom urethral stricture disease is thought to be unlikely and those patients with a possible neurological basis for their LUTS. In the younger patient presenting with LUTS (e.g. a man aged 20 to 40 or thereabouts) urethral stricture disease is a not uncommon cause of LUTS and BOO. Here, pressure–flow studies, while useful in determining the presence of obstruction, do not confirm its cause, and a simple retrograde urethrogram is in fact the only investigation that is required (*Fig. 4.2*). In any case, any attempt at performing pressure–flow studies is unlikely to succeed if the stricture is narrow, because a urethral catheter will prove impossible to insert.

It is sensible to measure **serum creatinine** in individuals with suspected BOO, given the potential for its effect on renal function – high bladder pressures can lead to high intrarenal pressures. **Urinalysis** or microscopy/culture are also valuable, and may identify patients with urinary tract infection or those with microscopic or dipstick haematuria. Patients with haematuria require cystoscopic examination of the bladder. **Serum PSA** testing is recommended in patients with LUTS, since the diagnosis of prostate cancer could alter the way the patient is managed.

Treatment of suspected BOO

Treatment of a patient with suspected BOO is dependent on the patient's presentation – LUTS or urinary retention.

Some patients may not want any specific treatment, once they have been reassured that it is unlikely that they have prostate cancer and that their risk of subsequent urinary retention is low. Studies of the natural history of LUTS (i.e. in the absence of treatment) suggest that, at least over a 5-year period of follow-up, one third of patients will experience worsening LUTS, in another third their

Fig. 4.2:
(a) A normal retrograde urethrogram. (b) A retrograde urethrogram showing a stricture in the bulbar urethra. Note the catheter, with balloon inflated in the distal end of the urethra (top left hand corner of picture). A thin 'tail' of contrast can be seen passing through the stricture at the bottom right hand corner of the picture.

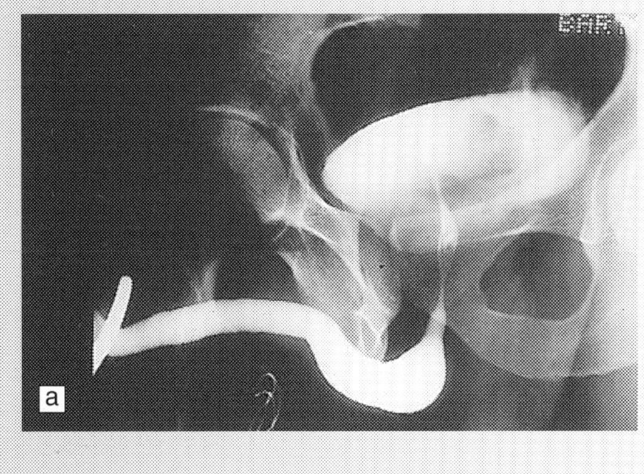

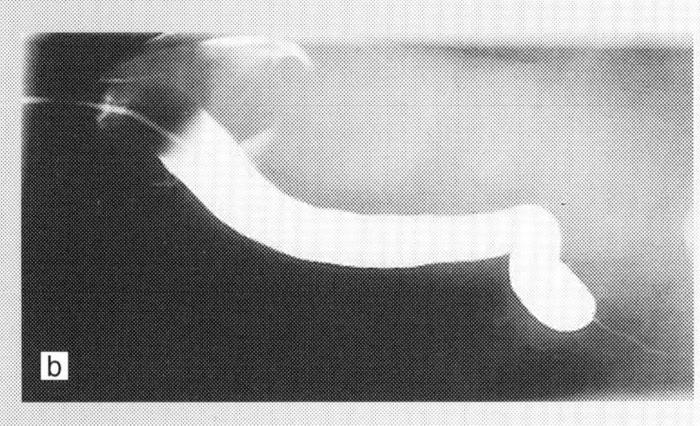

symptoms will remain unchanged, and in a further third there may be some improvement. For many patients this is reassuring. Others are simply not bothered by their symptoms even though they may 'score' quite high on a symptom score.

In those who wish to have some treatment a trial of an alpha-adrenergic blocking drug or a prostate-shrinking drug (e.g. finasteride) is worthwhile. The rationale behind using alpha-adrenergic blocking drugs ('alpha blockers') in men with BPH and LUTS is the presence of large quantities of smooth muscle in the prostatic stroma in BPH. It is thought that the tone of this smooth muscle may be an important factor in causing obstruction in BPH. While the improvement in flow rate with apha blockers is minimal (1–3 ml s^{-1} at most), they have nonetheless been shown, in randomized, placebo-controlled studies, to improve symptoms in a large proportion of men. Side-effects associated with alpha blocker medication include tiredness, dizziness and postural hypotension, though the newer selective agents (alfuzosin, terazosin, doxazosin and tamsulosin) are usually well tolerated.

Finasteride is an inhibitor of 5-alpha reductase, the enzyme responsible for conversion of testosterone to dihydrotestosterone (DHT), the active androgen in terms of prostatic growth and subsequent development of BPH. Prostate volume falls by approximately 20–30%, though it may take 6 months to have any impact on symptoms. Again, finasteride has been compared against placebo in large randomised studies, proving its effectiveness in the resolution of symptoms. It has a low side-effect profile, with approximately 5% of men reporting loss of libido and ejaculatory disturbance (Stoner et al., 1994).

If a trial of medical therapy has failed to improve a patient's symptoms, then one can consider transurethral prostatectomy (TURP). While not a major operation this is certainly not a minor one. The patient should be warned that the likelihood of symptom resolution is in the order of 60 to 70% and that serious complications, though relatively unusual, can occur. Approximately 3% of men will experience urinary sepsis, require a blood transfusion or need to return to the operating theatre for control of heavy bleeding. Less than 1% will develop permanent incontinence, but temporary urinary leakage, particularly that related to an urgent desire to void, is common after TURP. A total of 90% of men experience permanent retrograde ejaculation and 10% permanent loss of erection post-TURP. Rarely medical complications may occur (myocardial infarction, stroke, DVT). These factors need to be borne in mind when counselling a patient for TURP, and the patient will need to decide if their symptoms are bothersome enough to warrant the procedure.

Other treatment options for BPO include transurethral incision of the prostate (also known as bladder neck incision – BNI), laser prostatectomy (which involves resection or vaporization of the prostate by laser), and transurethral thermotherapy (transurethral application of microwave energy to the prostate which causes thermal damage to the obstructing prostatic tissue). Access to these treatments depends to an extent on local preferences and resources.

Patients with high-pressure chronic retention or high-pressure acute-on-chronic retention have high intrarenal pressures, and in the absence of adequate treatment of the cause of their BOO will develop progressive renal impairment. Here, the need for treatment in the form of prostatectomy (or long-term catheterization) is obvious.

In the case of patients with acute urinary retention or low-pressure acute-on-chronic retention, some urologists will almost always offer a trial without catheter or TWOC (also known as a trial of void, TOV), arguing that a significant proportion will void spontaneously and will not suffer a recurrence of retention. Others feel that the chance of further episodes of retention is high enough to warrant surgery without the need for attempts to remove the catheter, particularly if the patient has a history, prior to the episode of retention, of bothersome LUTS. It is certainly sensible to discuss the pros and cons of TWOC versus immediate surgery. It is also worth bearing in mind that acute urinary retention or low-pressure acute-on-chronic retention are sometimes precipitated by another acute event, such as an operation (hernia repair, hip replacement, back surgery such as laminectomy), acute illness or drug treatment (e.g. anticholinergic medication).

Additional treatments to improve the chances of a successful TWOC can be tried such as use of alpha-adrenergic blocking drugs or finasteride. The efficacy of these agents compared to placebo has not, as yet, been determined (trials are ongoing), but finasteride does seem to reduce the chances of acute retention in men with LUTS (McConnell et al., 1998) and it may well improve the chances of a successsful TWOC in those who have already presented with retention.

Patients with BPO presenting as recurrent acute retention, recurrent acute on chronic urinary retention or with high-pressure chronic retention have one of only two choices – a long-term indwelling catheter (or, rarely, clean intermittent self catheterization [ISC] if the patient is able and willing to do this) or a prostatectomy, which is usually a TURP, but occasionally an open prostatectomy. If the patient has an elevated creatinine or other problems which might cause problems with surgery or anaesthesia (uncontrolled hypertension, unstable ischaemic heart disease, clotting problems), then a period of time allowing the creatinine to stabilize and managing these medical problems is time well spent.

Urethral strictures

A urethral stricture is essentially a scar within the urethra. It can occur as a result of an inflammatory process or trauma. Historically, urethral strictures were often caused by gonococcal urethritis, which causes marked urethral scarring and hence stricture formation. This is now unusual with the rapid use of antibiotics for gonorrhoea. Nowadays, many strictures are caused by the trauma of urethral instrumentation by catheters or cystoscopes or occur months or years after transurethral resection of the prostate for BPO. Here the large-bore instruments used to resect the prostate can damage the lining of the urethra at sites distant from the prostatic urethra (the meatus and bulbar urethra being the most common sites of post-prostatectomy stricture). Pelvic fractures are often followed by urethral stricture formation. When there is complete urethral disruption a urethral stricture is inevitable. Prolonged urethral catheterization – even for just a few weeks – can lead to a stricture, and this is a classical scenario following coronary bypass graft surgery, where urethral ischaemia in a patient with cardiovascular disease may also be a factor. Finally, balanitis xerotica obliterans (BXO; also know as lichen sclerosis et atrophicus), an inflammatory condition affecting the glans penis and urethra, is the most common cause of strictures involving the urethra in the glans of the penis, though there may be more extensive involvement of the anterior urethra.

A carefully taken history may help identify the cause of the stricture. Examination of the penis may identify the characteristic diffuse white patches of BXO involving the meatus and fossa navicularis. In fact, the most common presentation of BXO is with phimosis – a hard, non-retractile foreskin which has lost its normal, supple texture. As mentioned above, retrograde urethrography allows radiologic visualization of the full extent of the stricture and this plays an important role in determining the type of subsequent treatment.

Urethral strictures may be treated by urethral dilatation, division of the stricture by a sharp knife under visual control (optical urethrotomy) or by formal open surgical repair (urethroplasty).

Urethral dilatation is a minor procedure which can be carried out under local anaesthetic, though many patients understandably prefer a spinal or general anaesthetic. However, overenthusiastic urethral dilatation or that which causes further trauma to the urethra (as evidenced by bleeding from the urethra) is likely in itself to cause further stricture formation which will require at the very least further dilatations. This may, however, be an acceptable method of management (though clearly not cure) of a stricture in an older man who wishes to avoid or is not fit enough for potentially major reconstructive surgery. Optical urethrotomy is a more controlled technique of dividing a urethral stricture and is a minimally invasive form of treatment, but it too is associated with a significant chance of subsequent restricturing. If a single optical urethrotomy fails to cure a stricture in a young man, then repeat urethrotomies are unlikely to be beneficial. ISC is proven to reduce the re-stricturing risk. Younger men may not be happy to accept the prospect of ISC, lifelong urethral dilatations or optical urethrotomies. In the young man with a stricture, serious consideration should be given to reconstructive surgery (urethroplasty). This may involve excision of the scarred length of urethra, with primary reanastomosis of healthy urethra to healthy urethra, or if the stricture is too long to allow this to be done, a flap of penile skin, or graft of buccal mucosa may be used to reconstruct the urethra.

BOO in women

The diagnosis of BOO in women relies on clinical suspicion – based on history and physical examination – supplemented by radiological and urodynamic investigations.

There is no consensus on the urodynamic definition of obstruction in women. Definitions based on Q_{max} alone, just as in men, cannot distinguish low flow due to detrusor hypocontractility from that due to BOO. Although voiding pressure is elevated in women with genuine BOO, severe obstruction as seen in some men is very unusual and the definitions of BOO based on pressure and flow that are used in men cannot be applied to women. Current definitions therefore use a combination of pressure and radiologic imaging of the bladder outlet at the time of voiding to diagnose BOO in women, and say that BOO is present if there is radiographic evidence of obstruction between the bladder neck and distal urethra in the presence of a sustained detrusor contraction (Nitti et al., 1999). This is usually associated with a low-flow rate, though not always. The key features of this definition are a focal area of urethral narrowing in the presence of a sustained bladder contraction. Impaired detrusor contractility can be defined as an unsustained contraction or a contraction inadequate to produce a normal flow rate or complete bladder emptying in the absence of a visualized, focal area of obstruction in the urethra.

Retention in women

Urinary retention in women has a broader range of potential causes than in men. A useful starting point for categorizing the causes of retention in women is to separate these into neurological and non-neurological. Neurologic causes include diabetes, multiple sclerosis, spinal cord pathology (spinal injury, spinal tumours, spondylolithesis), cerebrovascular accidents and transverse myelitis. Non-neurologic causes include various causes of urethral obstruction such as cystocele (a prolapsing bladder which impinges on, and therefore obstructs the urethra), rectocele or uterine prolapse, urethral stricture or pelvic masses of one sort or another (ovarian cysts, fibroid uterus), previous anti-incontinence surgery, genital herpes, and previous total abdominal hysterectomy. The latter probably causes retention by damaging the nerve supply to the detrusor and could therefore be defined as a neurological cause. Simple urinary infection can sometimes cause retention.

Prolonged epidural anaesthesia (e.g. during labour which ends in caesarian section, where the epidural is continued for some days) is a potent cause of retention in women. The bladder is usually catheterized in this situation, but a patient who fails to void after epidural anaesthesia should be carefully examined for the presence of bladder distension. Prolonged bladder distension can cause a so-called distension injury to the bladder, leading to subsequent impaired detrusor contractility and permanent problems with bladder drainage.

The various neurological conditions noted above usually cause retention due to detrusor failure. Indeed, this is the commonest cause of retention in women, urethral obstruction being relatively rare. Urinary retention is sometimes the first manifestation of multiple sclerosis in a woman, though MS more commonly causes detrusor hyperreflexia (leading to uncontrollable incontinence) than detrusor hyporeflexia (detrusor failure – leading to retention). As mentioned above a proportion of women with urethral obstruction show abnormal activity in the external sphincter on EMG recording, and it is thought that this may lead to inadequate relaxation of the sphincter during attempted voiding, sometimes causing retention (Fowler and Kirby 1986).

Urodynamic studies, which measure detrusor pressure (and therefore allow a diagnosis of detrusor failure to be confirmed) are useful in distinguishing detrusor failure from urethral obstruction as the cause of retention. Those patients with evidence of a normally contracting detrusor are likely to have urethral obstruction and if clinical pelvic examination and a pelvic ultrasound fail to identify a cystocele or pelvic mass as the cause of this, then a urethral stricture may well be the cause. In this situation urethral dilatation may be helpful. Unfortunately the only way of managing retention due to detrusor failure is to teach the patient how to perform intermittent self catheterization (or resort to long-term suprapubic catheterization) so that they can mechanically empty their bladder. Unfortunately cholinergic agonists have not proved useful in women who retain large residual urine volumes.

Key points

- The cause of BOO in an individual patient is dependent on the age of the patient. In older males BPO due to BPE is the commonest cause of BOO.
- There are two main ways in which BOO may present – retention or LUTS. Rarer presentations are renal failure and bladder stones.
- We no longer talk about 'prostatism' and instead use the term LUTS to avoid implying the cause of symptoms, which is not always the prostate.
- Urodynamic measurements (flow rate, residual urine volume, pressure–flow studies) have a limited capacity to predict outcome of treatment.
- Options for management of an elderly man with LUTS and a benign feeling prostate include watchful waiting, medical therapy (with alpha blockers or finasteride) or surgery such as TURP.

Cases

1. A 70-year-old man with no significant medical history presents with a 9 month history of LUTS (poor flow, hesitancy, nocturia twice per night). He has a benign feeling prostate and a PSA of 2 ng ml^{-1}.
   (a) Which investigations would you arrange?
   (b) What treatment would you initially recommend?

2. A 50-year-old man presents with a 4 month history of marked urgency, frequency and nocturia, passing urine 20 times during the day and 4 times at night. Urine culture has shown no infection and empirical treatment with antibiotics has failed to help.
   (a) Which questions would you specifically ask him and what particular points in examination would you look for?
   (b) Which investigations should be done?

3. A 45-year-old woman presents with urinary retention.
   (a) Which features on examination should you specifically look for?
   (b) Which investigations may be helpful in determining the cause?

Answers

1. (a) He should complete an AUA symptoms score to document the level of symptoms and in particular the degree of 'bother' he experiences from them. Blood should be sent for measurement of serum creatinine and urine for microscopy and culture. Measurement of his flow rate provides an objective assessment of lower urinary tract function, though it is debatable whether this has any major diagnostic or prognostic value.
   (b) If he is bothered by his symptoms and wants some form of treatment then a trial of medical therapy, with an alpha blocker or finasteride is the first-line of therapy.

2. (a) A young man with such symptoms may have underying bladder cancer, or more rarely a neurological basis for his symptoms. He should be specifically questioned about the presence of haematuria, bladder (suprapubic) pain and the presence of any neurological symptoms. His prostate should be examined, as such symptoms may sometimes be due to prostate cancer (firm, asymmetrical feeling prostate) or prostatitis (tenderness). A focused neurological examination should be performed.
   (b) His urine should be stick tested for the presence of blood and sent for microscopy, culture and cytology. Persistence of such symptoms warrants further investigation by flexible cystoscopy. If these are normal then formal urodynamic studies (pressure–flow studies with X-ray screening of the bladder and urethra during bladder filling and subsequent micturition) should be done.

3. (a) Once the bladder has been decompressed by catheterization the patient should undergo abdominal and pelvic examination (looking for the presence of abdominal and pelvic masses), examination of the perineum (for the presence of a cystocele, uterine prolapse or rectocele), and a focused neurological examination (power and reflexes in the legs and feet, perianal and pericoccygeal sensation).
   (b) A pelvic ultrasound may identify an ovarian mass or fibroid uterus, which can cause retention by compressing the urethra. Urodynamic testing (where bladder pressure is recorded during filling and voiding) can distinguish between detrusor failure (where detrusor pressure remains near zero during attempted voiding) and urethral obstruction (where no flow occurs despite a rise in detrusor pressure).

References

Abrams P. New words for old: lower urinary tract symptoms for "prostatism". *BMJ* 1994; **308**: 929–930.

Bruskewitz R.C., Reda D.J., Wasson J.H. et al. Testing to predict outcome after transurethral resection of the prostate. *J Urol* 1997; **157**: 1304–1308.

Fowler C.J., Kirby R.S. Electromyography of urethral sphincter in women with acute urinary retention. *Lancet* 1986; **1**: 1455 1457.

Griffiths D., Hofner K., van Mastrigt R. et al. Standardisation of terminology of lower urinary tract function: pressure-flow studies of voiding, urethral resistance and urethral obstruction. *Neurourol Urodyn* 1997; **16**: 1–18.

McConnell J.D., Barry M.J., Bruskewitz R.C. et al. Benign prostatic hyperplasia: diagnosis and treatment. *Clinical Practice Guideline No. 8*. AHCPR Publ. 94-0582, 1994, Agency for Healthcare Policy and Research, Rockville, MD.

McConnell J.D., Bruskewitz R., Walsh P. et al. The effect of finasteride on the risk of acute urinary retention and the need for surgical treatment among men with benign prostatic hyperplasia. *N Engl J Med* 1998; **338**: 557–563.

Neal D.E., Ramsden P.D., Sharples L. et al. Outcome of elective prostatectomy. *Br Med J* 1989; 299: 762–767.

Nitti V.W., Mai Tu L., Gitlin J. Diagnosing bladder outlet obstruction in women. *J Urol* 1999; **161**: 1535–1540.

Reynard J.M., Yang Q., Donovan J.L. et al. The ICS-'BPH' Study: uroflowmetry, lower urinary tract symptoms and bladder outlet obstruction. *Br J Urol* 1998; **82**: 619–623.

Stoner E. and Members of the Finasteride Study Group. Three-year safety and efficacy data on the use of finasteride in the treatment of benign prostatic hyperplasia. *Urology* 1994; **43**: 284–294.

CHAPTER 5

Urinary incontinence and catheters

Introduction

Urinary incontinence may be defined as an involuntary loss of urine whilst trying to inhibit micturition but may present in many different forms. Prevalent in all ages, it is an unpleasant symptom for the individual and carries a great social and psychological burden. Incontinence has a significant effect on partners and the family of the patient and represents an increasing draw on health resources for society as a whole. The incidence of urinary incontinence increases with age and it is estimated to affect up to 30% of elderly individuals in the community and 50% in institutions. The cost of care of a patient suffering from urinary incontinence not only relates to the cost of appliances, washing etc. but also to the treatment of co-existing medical complications including perineal rashes, pressure sores and urinary tract infection. Patients often become depressed and isolated and are more likely to require institutionalized care than similarly aged patients who are not affected. Despite these factors the care of patients with urinary incontinence has been sadly neglected. Patients rarely seek medical advice and when they do treatment is often inadequate and misdirected.

In order to effectively evaluate and treat patients presenting with urinary incontinence the clinician must have a sound understanding of the pathophysiology of the lower urinary tract and be conversant with treatment options available. Simple conservative measures are often adequate to provide significant benefit in patients especially when elderly but occasionally more intricate intervention is appropriate in carefully selected patients. This chapter reviews the pathophysiology of lower urinary tract dysfunction in relation to urinary incontinence and discusses current investigative techniques and treatment options.

The pathophysiology of the lower urinary tract with regard to urinary incontinence

The human lower urinary tract can be considered to consist of three distinct physiological parts, a reservoir or the bladder itself, a pump or the detrusor muscle and a valve mechanism for control of continence, the urinary sphincter. All three may coexist and interact anatomically and functionally but each may equally be involved in lower urinary tract dysfunction causing urinary incontinence.

The lower urinary tract is autonomically innervated by parasympathetic nerves (S2–S4), sympathetic nerves (T10–L2) and somatic or voluntary nerves (S2–S4). During filling the bladder stores urine at low pressures allowing the kidneys to continue to produce urine. The sphincteric mechanism remains closed providing urinary continence. The detrusor muscle itself actively relaxes during bladder filling, a property called dynamic compliance. The mechanism by which the detrusor achieves this is poorly understood but interaction between the sympathetic and parasympathetic innervation is undoubtedly important in this process. As maximum bladder capacity is reached (400 ml–500 ml) at a socially convenient time and place voiding is initiated by an initial fall in urethral and sphincteric activity followed by a coordinated detrusor contraction. Voiding is initiated by parasympathetic activity and simultaneous inhibition of sympathetic activity in the smooth muscle of the outlet of the bladder. When considering that the autonomic process of bladder filling and voiding is ultimately under voluntary control then it is no wonder that many pathological processes may interfere with this complex interaction and result in urinary incontinence.

The association between ageing and urinary incontinence is difficult to explain. Several changes in the lower urinary tract are noted as patients get older but none in isolation can be held responsible for the development of urinary incontinence. Functional bladder capacity is reduced as is the ability to suppress unwanted detrusor contractions during filling. Post-void residual volumes increase and urinary flow rates reduce but neither of these is likely to result in urinary incontinence. Elderly patients often excrete the bulk of their fluid intake at night-time and although this phenomenon may be exacerbated by heart disease, renal disease and in men bladder outflow obstruction secondary to prostate disease it rarely is sufficient to result in urinary incontinence.

In the younger patient there will almost invariably be a clear-cut cause for the onset of incontinence. In the elderly a minor event may be sufficient to render the patient incontinent in the presence of some or indeed all of these factors and consequently simple therapeutic measures may be all that is required to establish reasonable urinary control once more.

Clinical presentation

The presenting symptom of urinary incontinence may be obvious to both the patient and clinician but it is vitally important to get as much information as to the nature of the urinary incontinence, of its time onset and associated urinary symptoms.

Firstly it is important to ascertain whether the incontinence is a longstanding or transient phenomenon. Transient urinary incontinence may be related to a treatable isolated event the causes of which are listed in *Table 5.1*.

Table 5.1: Causes of transient incontinence

Causes of transient incontinence
Drugs e.g. sedatives, anticholinergics etc.
Constipation with stool impaction
Acute confusional state
Impaired mobility
Urinary tract infection
Atrophic vaginitis
Increased urine output e.g. heart failure, diuretics, hyperglycaemia etc.
Psychological dysfunction

Urinary incontinence may be associated with extreme urgency and other filling lower urinary tract symptoms, so-called **urge incontinence**. This type of incontinence is often associated with detrusor instability, other bladder disorders and occasionally is the presenting feature of neurological disease. **Stress urinary incontinence** is used to describe leakage of urine when intra-abdominal pressure is raised e.g. coughing or sneezing. It is commonly found in women who have given birth to children but is also seen occasionally in men following pelvic trauma or surgery where there has been some disruption to the urethral sphincter mechanism. **Overflow incontinence** is usually identified in men with chronic painless urinary retention (*Fig. 5.1*) but can occasionally occur in women. Patients will describe a continual loss of urine both during the day and night and may also be aware of a pelvic mass or fullness in the lower abdomen. **Continuous incontinence** may occur when there has been damage to the urethral sphincter mechanism or where urinary leakage bypasses the sphincter mechanism, e.g. a vesico-vaginal fistula. Clearly a recent history of urethral or pelvic surgery should raise the suspicion that iatrogenic injury to the lower urinary tract may have occurred.

In addition to a detailed history of the type of incontinence it is vital that an accurate history of associated **filling and voiding urinary symptoms** is taken. Associated symptoms related to the **gastrointestinal tract** e.g. constipation and a **gynaecological/obstetric history** should also be taken. The presence of any co-existent **neurological symptoms** may be relevant along with a **drug history** and details of any **previous surgery**. It should also be noted that herniated intervertebral discs and laminectomies below L1, where the spinal cord terminates, could be associated with poor detrusor function and lead to overflow incontinence on occasions.

General examination should include a search for specific **neurological abnormalities** e.g.

Fig. 5.1:
A 74-year-old man with overflow incontinence secondary to chronic urinary retention.

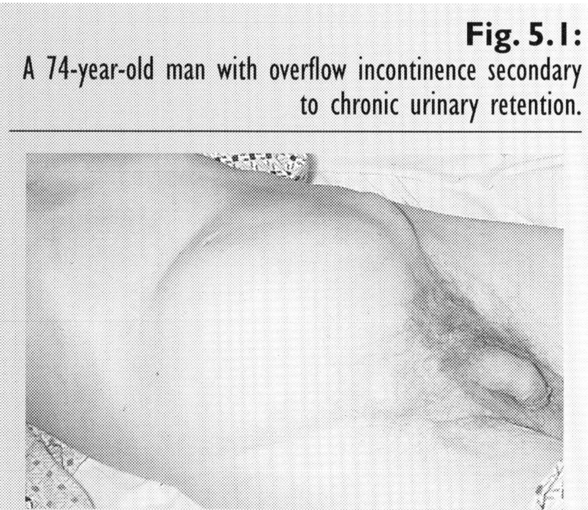

Table 5.2:
Investigations for urinary incontinence

Simple	Complex
Urinalysis	Cystometry (pressure–flow study)
Frequency/volume chart	Videocystometrogram
Pad testing	Neurophysiological tests
Urinary tract ultrasound	
Uroflowmetry	
Cystoscopy	

Parkinson's disease and the presence of other co-existent medical diseases e.g. congestive cardiac failure, peripheral oedema that may have an impact on diurnal urine production as previously discussed. Specific examination should identify abnormalities of the lower urinary tract. Unfortunately physical signs, except for the presence of a **palpable bladder** after voiding indicative of **chronic urinary retention**, are rarely evident. Pelvic examination in the female and rectal examination in the male may identify the presence of a **pelvic mass** arising from the lower gastrointestinal tract or gynaecological organs, including **atrophic vaginitis** and of course will allow the **prostate gland** to be palpated. **Stress leakage** during coughing can be demonstrated in females with clinical symptoms suggesting stress incontinence along with the degree of **bladder base descent**. The presence of a **cystocele** and/or **rectocele** should also be noted.

Investigations

Clinicians are often tempted to initiate complex investigations to study underlying lower urinary tract dysfunction in incontinent patients. These more complex tests are often not needed and may not contribute much in the way of further patient management. Details of these investigations are also discussed in Chapters 2 and 4, but their specific role in the management of urinary incontinence is outlined (*Table 5.2*).

Urinalysis should be performed to identify the presence of a urinary tract infection and to look for malignant cells on **cytology**: a bladder tumour may occasionally be the cause of incontinence in the absence of other lower urinary tract symptoms.

A most useful and frequently overlooked investigation is the **frequency/volume chart**. The patient or carer records the time and amount of each void throughout the day and night and episodes of incontinence are also noted. This chart provides a sense of purpose and reinforcement for the patient, objectively quantifies the severity of the incontinence and in more complex cases provides valuable clues as to the underlying diagnosis. Patients who are incontinent at night in the supine position but dry whilst sleeping in a chair during the day may have a postural diuresis related to heart failure. A patient who is wet during the morning but dry afterwards may be suffering from incontinence precipitated by diuretic therapy that may be improved by increasing the frequency of visits to the lavatory. **Pad testing** can also objectively measure the degree of urine loss and may be especially useful when the perceived severity of symptoms does not tally with the observed clinical assessment.

An **ultrasound scan (USS)** both before and after micturition is mandatory in incontinent patients. In those with significant post-micturition residuals the upper tracts should also be scanned to look for the presence of hydronephrosis. In those patients with evidence of microscopic haematuria, abnormal urine cytology or marked filling lower urinary tract symptoms a **cystoscopy** must be undertaken to rule out the possibility of a bladder tumour being present. Many clinicians perform cysto-urethroscopy as a matter of course in the assessment of the incontinent patient especially when surgical treatment is being contemplated. **Intravenous urography** is indicated where trauma to the ureter is suspected following pelvic surgery and the presence of a fistula is being investigated. A **cystogram** may be useful for confirming the clinical diagnosis of a vesico-vaginal fistula.

Videocystometrography (VCMG) has the ability to both define functional and anatomical evidence of lower urinary tract dysfunction causing urinary incontinence and is thus the investigation of choice in patients who are likely to undergo surgical therapy.

Neurophysiological testing of urethral sphincter activity etc. is not used widely and rarely adds information that has not already been obtained using VCMG.

Treatment

The importance of defining the underlying abnormality in lower urinary tract dysfunction before initiating 'blind' treatment cannot be overemphasized. Repeated failure of treatment leads to rapid demoralization and depression and a belief that no remedy is going to be of any value. The basic pathophysiology of urinary incontinence can be summarized as follows (*Table 5.3*).

Table 5.3: Pathophysiology of urinary incontinence

Overactive detrusor activity during filling
Underactive detrusor activity during voiding
Genuine stress incontinence
Bladder outlet obstruction
Lower urinary tract fistulae (e.g. vesico-vaginal)

Detrusor overactivity will often respond to specific **bladder training exercises** or prompted voiding regimes. Where a cause of an unstable detrusor can be identified e.g. in association with bladder outflow obstruction then correction of the underlying problem will often result in an improvement in detrusor function. If these measures fail then supplementing bladder training with **bladder suppressant medication** may be indicated. Drugs exhibiting anti-cholinergic activity e.g. oxybutynin, tolteradine are frequently successful in improving symptoms. Side effects, e.g. dry mouth, are often troublesome, however. Patients who are resistant to pharmacotherapy may be carefully considered for surgical therapy. **Distension of the bladder** under general anaesthetic is occasionally utilized but rarely results in sustained benefit. Augmentation of the bladder by **detrusor myomectomy** or '**clam ileocystoplasty**' can produce excellent results in the more severely affected younger patient.

Poor bladder contraction (**detrusor failure**) may result in urinary incontinence and is often irreversible. Initially, especially if there has been a distension injury to the bladder, a **period of catheterization** will 'rest' the bladder and a trial of voiding will result in better bladder emptying. Unfortunately this is not always the case and therapeutic trials with **alpha-adrenergic blockers** to reduce bladder outlet resistance or **cholinergic drugs** to promote detrusor contraction are rarely useful. **Intermittent** or **permanent catheterization** of the bladder is then indicated.

Genuine stress incontinence is prevalent in women after childbirth and is initially treated with **conservative measures** such as weight loss and instruction in **pelvic floor exercises**. Surgery is offered to those with severe symptoms who have not responded to these measures and consists of **elevation of the bladder neck** at either endoscopic or open operation. In men and women where the urethral sphincter mechanism is thought to be deficient then periurethral injection of bulking agents may improve symptoms.

Relief of **bladder outflow obstruction** in males (prostate or bladder neck) and females (urethra) using relevant surgical techniques will often improve urinary incontinence but patients should be carefully counselled as to the outcomes of such procedures which are not always successful in treating this symptom in isolation.

Lower urinary tract fistulae usually require reconstruction at open operation but occasionally uretero-vaginal fistulae will heal spontaneously with the aid of an indwelling double J stent.

It should be remembered that although treatment for urinary incontinence is often successful at improving symptoms, complete continence might not be achieved. Patients should be clearly advised regarding outcomes of treatment so that unrealistic expectations of 'cure' are not inferred. In complex cases where treatment options have repeatedly failed the use of an **artificial urinary sphincter** is sometimes appropriate. Ultimately **permanent catheterization** or **urinary diversion** may be suitable treatment options in those severely incapacitated by their incontinence.

Urinary catheters

Catheterization of the lower urinary tract has been performed by man for centuries in an effort to relieve urinary retention. The ancient Egyptians made urinary catheters from papyrus and in Victorian times men would carry short metal catheters in their top hats to relieve lower urinary tract symptoms. Whereas retention of urine historically would often result in death, nowadays a wide variety of catheters are available to relieve urinary retention both on a permanent and intermittent basis.

A catheter may be introduced into the bladder via a suprapubic or urethral route. Urethral catheters are based around a common design but vary in size, channel number and manufacturing compound. The indications, technique and complications of suprapubic catheterization are discussed in Chapter 3, page 16.

Catheters were previously made of either red rubber or gum elastic but it became evident that these caused extreme irritation to the urethral mucosa and have thus become obsolete. The more modern catheter is usually made of a plastic or latex compound although silastic catheters are virtually non-irritant and should be used for patients who require long-term catheter drainage or are immediately recovering from urethral or bladder reconstructive surgery.

The urethral catheter has been designed to drain either urine or blood from the urinary bladder. Urine will drain freely through a tiny diameter hole near or at the end of the catheter whereas blood requires a wider bore channel with a large hole or multiple holes to minimize obstruction to flow through the catheter with clot. Haematuria catheters possess an additional channel to allow irrigation of the bladder to prevent further clot formation and are often referred to as **irrigation catheters** (*Fig. 3.1*). Occasionally in a man with a large prostate it is difficult to pass a catheter through the prostatic urethra and therefore a bend at the neck of the catheter (**coude**) has been developed to overcome this difficulty. When a catheter is left in the bladder for several days then a small balloon is inflated at the end of the catheter so that it can be retained in the bladder without the need for sutures etc. This is known as a **Foley catheter**.

Complications of urethral catheters include urethral trauma and development of 'false passage' or stricture, UTI or septicaemia, urethral erosion (acquired hypospadias), blockages by debris, haematuria, stone formation, chronic cystitis and possibly squamous carcinoma of the bladder.

In general terms if a patient is being catheterized for urinary retention then the smallest catheter that will perform the task is ideal e.g. a 14 F Foley catheter. Occasionally a larger and therefore slightly stiffer catheter is required to negotiate the prostatic urethra in the male and if long-term drainage is required then the catheter should be made of silastic. If the bladder is full of blood or bleeding is to be expected e.g. after prostatic surgery then a large (20 F–24 F) irrigating catheter should be inserted. Great care must always be taken when introducing a urethral catheter, especially in male patients, as the urethra is easily traumatized. If resistance can be felt during attempted catheterization then it is safer to ask for specialist help from a urologist or insert a suprapubic catheter. The use of a catheter introducer should be avoided if at all possible.

Key points

- Urinary incontinence is extremely prevalent and is a huge drain on health resources.
- Many patients never seek medical advice.
- An understanding of the pathophysiology of the lower urinary tract is essential before advising individual patients.
- Always be aware that incontinence may be a presenting feature of neurological or cardiovascular disease.
- Always ask the patient to produce a frequency/volume chart.
- Complex urodynamic tests are not always indicated.

Cases

1. A 37-year-old woman presents with a history of leaking urine during her exercise classes. She has had three children, the last requiring a forceps delivery.
   (a) Which investigations would you perform?
   (b) How would you treat her in the first instant?
   (c) What would you do if this treatment failed?

2. A 28-year-old woman has been continually wet following a vaginal hysterectomy.
   (a) What is the most likely diagnosis?
   (b) How would you confirm the diagnosis?
   (c) How would you treat this problem?

3. A 74-year-old man has mixed urge and dribbling incontinence following a TURP. The possible causes of his incontinence include detrusor instability, residual bladder outflow obstruction and sphincter damage/weakness.
   (a) How would you investigate this man?
   (b) How would you treat each of these possible causes?

Answers

1. (a) Urinalysis, an ultrasound scan of her bladder before and after micturition, cystoscopy?
   (b) Advice regarding weight loss etc. and instruction by specialist in pelvic floor exercises.
   (c) Consider a videourodynamic study prior to surgical intervention.
2. (a) A vesico-vaginal fistula.
   (b) Clinical examination may reveal an indurated area over the anterior wall of the vagina, a cystogram will demonstrate a leak from the bladder with contrast pooling in the vagina and a cystoscopy will reveal the fistula usually over the posterior surface of the bladder at or near the midline.
   (c) Initially a catheter is inserted into the bladder to control the urinary incontinence. Occasionally the fistula will heal after about three weeks of permanent catheterization but usually open repair of the fistula is required.
3. (a) Urinalysis to look for urinary tract infection, Ultrasound scan of bladder to look for residual urine post-micturition, uroflowmetry, videocystometrogram, cystoscopy.
   (b) Detrusor instability: bladder training, anticholinergics medication. Residual bladder outflow obstruction: further prostatic surgery. Sphincter damage/weakness: submucosal bulking agents to sphincter active area, artificial urinary sphincter.

Further reading

Gillenwater J., Grayhack J.T., Howards S.S. and Duckett J.W. (1996). *Adult and Paediatric Urology*. Third ed. Mosby, St. Louis.

Walsh P.C., Retik A.B., Stamey T.A. and Vaughan E.D. (1999). *Campbell's Urology*. Seventh ed. Saunders, Philadelphia.

Whitfield H.N., Hendry W.F., Kirby R.S. and Duckett J.W. (1998). *Textbook of Genitourinary Surgery*. Second ed. Blackwell Science, Oxford.

CHAPTER 6

The neuropathic bladder

The neuropathic (neurogenic) bladder may be defined simply as one whose function is disturbed by neurological disease affecting the nerve supply of the bladder. An aura of perceived mystery surrounds the neuropathic bladder, but as with all seemingly complex problems the fundamentals of the neuropathic bladder can be broken down into a few simple rules. In reality, the management of the neuro-pathic bladder is relatively straightforward, though this should not be taken to imply that treatment is necessarily always successful.

Pathophysiology

It is not possible to understand the pathophysiology of the neuropathic bladder without understanding normal bladder and urethral function and without having some idea about the innervation of the bladder and urethra.

The bladder has both a motor and sensory nerve supply. The **motor** supply of the bladder is derived from the autonomic nervous system and is principally **parasympathetic** (*Fig. 6.1*). The parasympathetic nerve cells supplying the bladder originate in the intermediolateral cell column of S2, 3 and 4. The preganglionic nerve fibres are conveyed to the bladder in the pelvic nerves and they synapse with postganglionic nerve cells in the pelvic plexus and also on the surface of the bladder. The motor supply of the **trigone and lower ureters is sympathetic** (T10–L2).

The **sensory** supply of the bladder is transmitted in both **parasympathetic** nerves (stretch, fullness, pain) and **sympathetic** nerves (pain, touch, temperature).

The **urethral sphincter** has both striated and smooth muscle components. The striated muscle of the urethral sphincter is known as the intrinsic rhabdosphincter. The **striated sphincter muscle** receives its motor supply from **somatic** nerves (not

Fig. 6.1:
Motor nerve supply of the bladder. This is principally parasympathetic, from S2–4, the nerves being transmitted from the cord to the bladder in pelvic nerves. The trigone and lower ureters are innervated by sympathetic nerves derived from T10–L2.

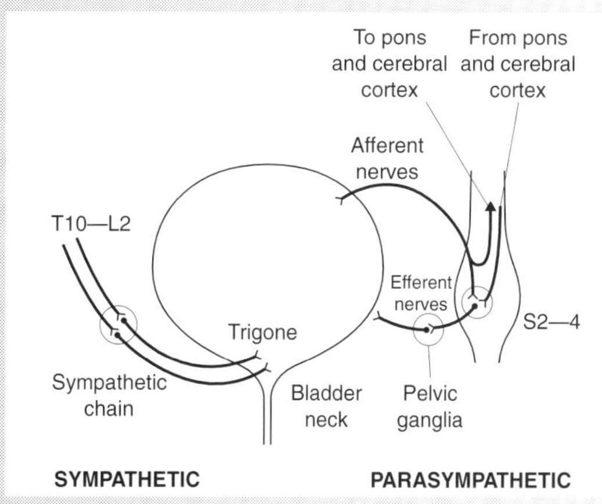

parasympathetic), derived from S2–4 (from a region called Onuf's nucleus in the sacral cord) and transmitted to the urethra in the pudendal nerves. The **smooth muscle sphincter**, at the bladder neck, is innervated by **sympathetic nerves**. Their cell bodies lie in T10–L2 spinal segments and travel to the bladder neck in the hypogastric nerves (*Fig. 6.2*).

In terms of normal function the bladder is designed to store large volumes of urine at low pressure, and without much sensation of bladder filling or desire to void, until the bladder is relatively full. At this point the desire to pass urine becomes strong, but this urge can be suppressed until there is an appropriately convenient time to void. During micturition the bladder contracts, accompanied at the same time by a coordinated

Fig. 6.2:
The innervation of the urethral sphincter. The striated sphincter muscle is innervated by somatic fibres (*not* parasympathetic or sympathetic) derived from S2–4. These nerve fibres are transmitted to the sphincter in the pudendal nerves. The smooth muscle component of the urethral sphincter (the bladder neck) is innervated by sympathetic neurons whose cell bodies lie in T10–L2, and they are transmitted to the bladder neck in the hypogastric nerves.

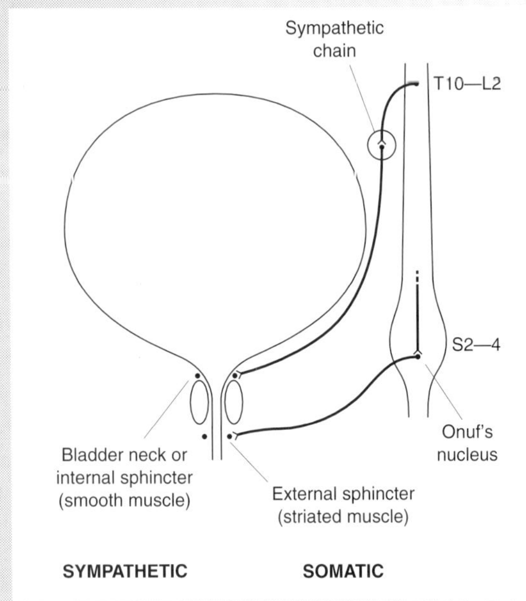

relaxation of the bladder neck and external urethral sphincter, so allowing the unobstructed flow of urine through the urethra, until the bladder is empty. Thus, bladder and sphincter contraction have a reciprocal relationship, such that when the bladder is relaxed the sphincter is contracted (during bladder filling) and continence is maintained. Conversely, when the bladder contracts, the sphincter relaxes (during micturition) for a sufficient time to allow complete bladder emptying to occur. There are many causes of the neuropathic bladder, but they all affect to some degree or other the fundamental functions of urine storage by the bladder and/or urine conduction by the urethra.

The centre for coordinating bladder and urethral function lies within the pons and is known as the pontine micturition centre. The cell bodies of parasympathetic motor fibres (S2–4) innervating the bladder muscle and somatic motor fibres (S2–4) innervating the striated urethral sphincter are located in the sacral cord and they receive descending inputs from the **pontine micturition centre**. The pontine micturition centre is responsible for ensuring that the activity of the bladder and urethral sphincter are coordinated so that one contracts while the other relaxes.

Patients with neurological conditions affecting lower urinary tract function may have an overactive or underactive bladder, an overactive or underactive sphincter or any combination of bladder over or underactivity with sphincter over- or underactivity. The **balance** between bladder and sphincter function will determine **bladder pressure** and the **effectiveness of bladder emptying**, and these 2 factors – pressure and volume – will, in turn, influence the symptoms the patient is likely to experience and their risk of high intrarenal pressures and thus subsequent renal damage. Thus, whenever you see a patient with a neuropathic bladder, you should think 'how good is this patient's bladder at emptying?' and 'what is their bladder pressure?'.

The balance between bladder and sphincter function can, in simplistic terms, be thought of as leading to 3 types of bladder dysfunction – contractile, intermediate and acontractile (Mundy, 1988).

Contractile bladders can contract with sufficient strength and duration to produce bladder emptying as long as there is no associated bladder outlet obstruction. Bladder outlet obstruction can be due to an overactive sphincter. Patients in whom the pontine micturition centre has effectively been disconnected from the sacral spinal cord (the classic example being **spinal cord injury**) lose the coordination between bladder and urethral sphincter function and when their bladder contracts, so too does their urethral sphincter (the complete reverse of what should normally happen). This condition is known as detrusor-external sphincter dyssynergia or DESD (*Fig. 6.3*). Such patients have bladders that contract forcefully

Fig. 6.3:
Detrusor-external sphincter dyssynergia. This shows a voiding cystourethrogram – the patient is attempting to pass urine and the external sphincter (the narrowing seen in the urethra between the prostatic and bulbar urethra) continues to contract – at a time when it should be relaxing.

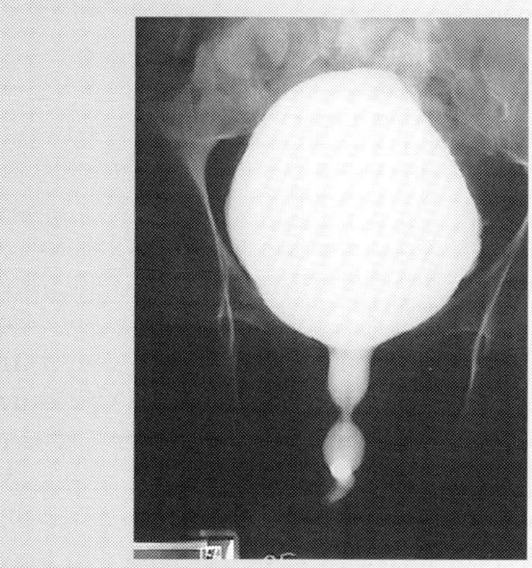

against a closed external sphincter. The end result is easy to predict. Their bladders do not empty completely, they develop very high bladder pressures and as a consequence they have high intrarenal pressures. Patients with lesions above the pons (e.g. cerebrovascular accidents [CVAs]) and therefore with an intact pons and an intact connection between the pons and the sacral cord, have no associated bladder outlet obstruction. Thus, their bladders are very overactive (hyperreflexic – just like hyperactive tendon reflexes and skeletal muscle spasticity), but their urethral sphincters have normal activity. As a consequence when their bladders develop a forceful contraction, their sphincter (which is normally functioning) cannot withstand the pressure that the bladder develops, and they leak. This is the situation in patients with CVAs above the pons.

Intermediate bladders exhibit contractile activity, but this is rather like the contraction of the atria in atrial fibrillation, and as a result no bladder contraction which is useful for bladder emptying is produced. Such bladders are often associated with a constantly active sphincter, which develops pressures higher than a normal sphincter. Its resistance is thus relatively high. As the bladder fills up the constant background level of bladder contraction, combined with an overactive sphincter leads to ever increasing bladder pressures. The bladder exhibits poor compliance by which we mean high pressures at low volumes (the reverse of the normal situation; normal bladders are highly compliant – and thus hold large volumes of urine at low pressure). As a consequence the kidneys may be at risk of high intrarenal pressures. Bladder pressure will eventually overcome the sphincter pressure and the patient leaks urine. Thus, such patients have a urethral sphincter that is both obstructive and incompetent. They have the worst of both worlds – a high risk of renal damage and incontinence.

Acontractile bladders show little or no activity and thus as the bladder fills the pressure remains low. The patient will thus retain urine, though at high bladder volumes the urethral sphincter will allow leakage of some urine. Effectively they have retention, with overflow incontinence at high volumes.

This classification system is simple, and it is this simplicity that makes it so useful. It is easy to remember and more importantly it tells you whether the kidneys are at risk, what you have to do to protect them, what the likely mechanism underlying the patient's incontinence is, and how to help the patient achieve continence. Everything centres around bladder **pressure** (is it high, is it low?) and bladder **volume** (is it high, is it low?) and often one can have a pretty good idea from the appearance of the kidneys and bladder on ultrasound as to what the bladder pressure is likely to be. For example, one can infer from bilateral hydronephrosis in the presence of a bladder containing several hundred millilitres of urine that the bladder is likely to be a high pressure one and that the sphincter is likely to be obstructive to some degree or other. If necessary, the exact urodynamic diagnosis can be confirmed by measurement of bladder pressure during bladder filling, and pressure and flow during micturition with simultaneous X-ray screening of the bladder and in particular the external sphincter and bladder neck (VCMG).

This system of classification – contractile, intermediate, acontractile – is a urodynamic one. Neuropathic bladders can also be thought of in terms of the level of the lesion causing them. Just as strokes and other neurological conditions affecting the motor side of the nervous system are described as being either upper motor neuron or lower motor neuron, so one can describe a neuropathic bladder as being an **upper motor neuron-type bladder** or a **lower motor neuron-type bladder**. This classification, based on the level of the lesion, can be useful because it is closely related (usually) to the type of bladder and urethral sphincter function that one can expect. An upper motor neuron lesion is a defect between the brain and the anterior horn cells of the spinal cord. Thus, any injury to the brain or spinal cord, as long as it is above the level of the sacral cord (where the motor neurons of the bladder and striated urethral sphincter reside), will result in an **upper motor neuron bladder** (and urethra). Lower motor neuron lesions represent defects between the anterior horn cells and the peripheral organ of innervation (the lower motor neuron cell bodies lie in the anterior horn). For example, damage to the pelvic nerves may occur during surgery to the rectum or uterus. Such lesions will lead to a **lower motor neuron-type bladder** (and urethra).

An upper motor neuron lesion results in hyperactive tendon reflexes and skeletal muscle spasticity. An 'upper motor neuron bladder' will be overactive, demonstrating either hyperreflexic contractions or a progressive rise in pressure during bladder filling. A lower motor neuron lesion causes loss of deep tendon reflexes and flaccidity of skeletal muscles. A 'lower motor neuron bladder' is underactive – the bladder simply fills up without any rise in pressure and when the patient tries to void their bladder fails to contract.

While this rule usually holds true, it does not always do so. Thus, some patients with cervical and thoracic spinal cord injuries (i.e. upper motor neuron lesions) have flaccid, acontractile bladders – the type of bladder one would normally expect to occur with a lower motor neuron lesion (Kaplan et al., 1996). It is this clinical observation that has led to the hypothesis that such cases might represent a combination of spinal injuries – the obvious upper motor neuron lesion of the cervical or thoracic spinal cord injury, combined with a covert sacral cord lesion. Any lesion damaging the sacral cord (and hence the cell bodies of the lower motor neurons) will result in a lower motor neuron lesion, and this prevents the upper motor neuron lesion from becoming manifest.

Whether a patient with a neuropathic bladder has urinary symptoms such as incontinence, or high intrarenal pressures which put them at risk of **renal failure**, will depend on the balance between bladder and sphincter activity. A patient with an overactive (hyper-reflexic) bladder and a weak sphincter will be wet, but their kidneys are not necessarily in danger because the high bladder pressures cause such a degree of leakage that they do not retain any significant volume of urine in their bladder. Patients with overactive bladders and overactive sphincters may develop such high bladder pressures that even their overactive sphincters cannot stop them from leaking, but in between leaking the constantly high bladder pressures lead to high intrarenal pressures and eventual renal failure. Those with active sphincters and low-pressure (underactive) bladders simply cannot void, at least at normal bladder volumes. Their bladders become very full, until the pressure is enough to overcome the sphincter pressure, at which point they leak. The pressures are not normally high enough to cause back pressure on their kidneys. Finally, those with weak sphincters and low-pressure bladders may retain moderate volumes of urine, but any added stress on their bladder (coughing, straining their abdominal wall muscles while transferring from a wheelchair) may be enough to make them leak.

The presence of residual urine after voiding or attempted voiding may lead to the development of recurrent urinary tract infections. Indeed, efficient antegrade flow of urine (i.e. complete bladder emptying) is a major factor in preventing most of us from developing urinary tract infections. Thus, if you are unable to efficiently empty your bladder you are at risk for the development of urinary infection.

There are, then, three essential problems that the neuropathic patient may face – urinary symptoms such as urgency and incontinence, the potential for high intrarenal pressures and thus subsequent renal failure, and the risk of recurrent urinary infection due to inefficient antegrade flow of urine. While incontinence can obviously be very bothersome, preservation of renal function is clearly a priority as is prevention of recurrent infections, which may be particularly damaging if they are associated with high bladder pressures and intrarenal reflux of infected urine.

In the longer term, patients with neuropathic bladders are also at risk of developing renal and bladder calculi. This is because they often have chronically infected urine, urinary stasis (inefficient antegrade flow of urine) and a degree of immobility which may lead to increased mobilization of bone calcium and hence hypercalciuria.

Investigation of the patient with a neuropathic bladder

Investigation of any patient with a neurological condition known to have a potential effect on bladder function is directed at assessing renal function by **serum creatinine** and imaging the kidneys and bladder by **ultrasound**, specifically looking for the presence of hydronephrosis and the presence and volume of any residual urine. This in itself may be all that is needed to allow a decision on subsequent management to be made. For example, high bladder residual urine volumes in the presence of hydronephrosis (with or without urine infection) are virtually diagnostic of high bladder pressures and bladder outlet obstruction. Such a situation indicates the need for improved bladder drainage, by for example, intermittent self-catheterization. If this improves renal function, results in resolution of the hydronephrosis on subsequent scanning, improves continence and stops or at least reduces the frequency of UTIs to a tolerable level, then nothing further needs to be done. No complex urodynamic tests are required. A **plain KUB X-ray** is warranted since many patients with neuropathic bladders have stones.

Persistent hydronephrosis or incontinence after the introduction of simple measures, will indicate the need for formal assessment of bladder and urethral function, by VCMG. This allows bladder pressure during filling and voiding to be measured, and allows visualization of the bladder and sphincter during voiding so allowing an assessment of sphincter function relative to bladder function. This allows a more rational approach to therapy.

If a more accurate measure of renal function is required, then **creatinine clearance** can be measured to give an indication of glomerular filtration rate and from a **MAG3 renogram** a measure of effective renal plasma flow can be derived and compared against the expected level for the patient's age, sex and weight.

Examining the patient who you think might have a neuropathic bladder

There may be times when you see a patient whose LUTS suggest an underlying neurological problem or who for some other reason you suspect might have a neurological condition which could affect bladder function.

From a neurological perspective the bladder and urethra are innervated by the lowest part of the spinal cord (by S2, 3 and 4). In this respect the bladder is said to be under the feet (which are innervated by L4 and 5 and S1 and 2). Thus, a lesion in the spinal cord affecting the feet is likely to involve the bladder as well.

Consider a neurological basis for a patient's LUTS if the patient reports neurological symptoms in their legs or feet (loss of power, tingling sensations, 'my legs just feel funny'); disturbance of bowel function; difficulty with obtaining or maintaining an erection; reduced volume of ejaculate or absence of ejaculation or of the sensation of orgasm; odd sensations in the penis or clitoris e.g. genital 'burning' sensations.

LUTS occurring in association with back pain should be taken seriously. We all experience back pain from time to time, but back pain which fails to resolve within a few weeks and which is progressive and relentless suggests the possibility of a disc lesion, spinal tumour or some other lesion. Interscapular pain suggests the possibility of a spinal tumour or metastases and is an indication for MRI of the spinal cord.

A focused neurological examination should include examination of power and tendon reflexes in the legs and feet, examination for loss of sensation in the legs, feet and perineum and testing for the presence of the bulbocavernosus reflex and for anal tone and contraction of the pelvic floor muscles.

The bulbocavernosus reflex (BCR) is a local sacral cord reflex which tests the integrity of the pudendal afferents, the sacral cord (segments S2–4) and the pudendal efferents. It is the reflex contraction of the striated muscles of the pelvic floor on stimulation of the glans or clitoris (it can also be elicited by gently pulling on a urethral catheter). The muscles which contract are bulbocavernosus and ischiocavernosus, the external anal sphincter and the external urethral sphincter. It can be elicited in the majority (98%) of neurologically intact males and in most (80%) neurologically intact females. Thus, in the male in particular (and usually in the female) its absence is very suggestive of a lesion in the conus medullaris (the conical end of the spinal cord where S2–4 lie) or cauda equina (the descending and ascending nerve roots which form the spinal nerves on exiting the vertebral foramina) or a more peripheral lesion. However, the presence of a normal BCR does not exclude such a lesion, so if you suspect a lesion in this area of the cord or in the cauda equina, get an MRI.

Sensory loss in the neuropathic bladder first manifests as loss of sensation in the pericoccygeal region (rather than the perianal region), so it is not enough to test just perianal sensation.

Treatment of the patient with a neuropathic bladder

Some aspects of treatment of the neuropathic bladder have already been discussed. The **aims of treatment** are to preserve renal function, achieve and maintain continence, and to prevent recurrent urinary tract infection and bladder and renal stone formation.

These aims can be achieved by lowering resting bladder pressure, ensuring efficient bladder emptying and, in cases where there is sphincter weakness, improving sphincter function.

Efficient bladder emptying reduces bladder pressure and so can prevent high intra-renal pressures. This can be achieved by clean intermittent self catheterization (ISC), indwelling bladder catheterization (usually suprapubic) or in males by dividing the external urethral sphincter if this is obstructive (so-called external sphincterotomy).

In the 1940s intermittent catheterization became one of the mainstays of management of the bladder in spinal injured neuropathic patients at Stoke Mandeville Hospital and it had a major impact on reducing urological morbidity and mortality in these patients. Lapides et al. (1972) introduced the concept of clean ISC, and it is fair to say that this has been a revolutionary method for improving bladder emptying in neuropathic patients, thereby lowering bladder pressures and so protecting the kidneys and improving continence. Clearly, in order to be able to perform ISC the patient must have good hand function, they must appreciate the rationale behind the technique and understand that they may have to catheterize themselves 7 or 8 times a day. They must also have a bladder which is able to hold a volume of urine (at not too high a pressure) which is high enough for them not to need to catheterize every hour or so. A patient who needs to perform ISC every hour would clearly spend a considerable amount of their day doing so and such a commitment in time and effort may simply not fit in with their lifestyle. This may be particularly so for the wheelchair bound patient who may need to transfer to a toilet to perform ISC.

The use of an indwelling urethral catheter can work very well for some patients. It obviously keeps the bladder completely empty, so maintaining bladder pressure at zero. Indwelling catheters are usually suprapubic to avoid the possible complication of urethral meatus erosion. While many patients with indwelling catheters do not get recurrent UTIs or catheter blockages from debris within the bladder, others do and this can be a major problem. There may be an increased risk of development of bladder cancer in the chronically catheterized bladder. For these reasons and because of altered body image many people do not like the concept of a chronic indwelling catheter.

An alternative method of achieving efficient bladder emptying in male patients who have lost the normal coordination between bladder contraction and external sphincter relaxation (DESD) is external sphincterotomy. DESD classically occurs in cervical or thoracic spinal cord injury or spina bifida. Division of the external sphincter is performed endoscopically and renders the obstructing external sphincter incompetent, so allowing efficient bladder emptying when the bladder contracts. A degree of continence is maintained if the bladder neck is still functioning, though often the patient will have to wear a condom sheath as they may have no or very little warning of when their bladder is going to reflexly empty, and if (as is usually the case) they are wheelchair-bound, it is simply more convenient to void into a sheath attached to a leg bag.

ISC alone may not, however, achieve adequate lowering of bladder pressure and anticholinergic drugs, which reduce contractility of the detrusor smooth muscle, may be necessary to increase effective bladder capacity. These anticholinergic drugs include oxybutynin, tolterodine, propiverine and flavoxate. In a high pressure bladder where a combination of anticholinergic medication and ISC has failed to reduce bladder pressure enough to result in a lowering of intrarenal pressure or to prevent incontinence because of high bladder pressures, one must resort either to an indwelling catheter or to an operative procedure designed to increase bladder capacity. In practice this usually means augmentation of bladder capacity by placing a patch of bowel (small or large intestine or both) into the bivalved bladder (so-called 'clam' cystoplasty because the bladder is opened up like a clam shell and the bowel patch is stitched onto the rim of bladder). Such bladders have a large capacity, but this is achieved at the expense of rendering any residual bladder contraction ineffective for achieving bladder emptying, so the patient may well have to perform ISC afterwards to empty their bladder. An alternative for increasing bladder capacity is autoaugmentation, where a disc of bladder muscle is removed from the dome of bladder and the intact underlying mucosa bulges outwards, the resulting diverticulum providing a small increase in capacity and reduction in pressure (*Fig. 6.4*).

Optimizing bladder emptying and lowering bladder pressure may be all that is required to achieve continence, but in patients who also have sphincter weakness and where anticholinergic

Fig. 6.4:
Autoaugmentation of the bladder. A disc of detrusor muscle has been carefully dissected off the dome of the bladder, allowing the (intact) underlying mucosa to bulge outwards, forming a diverticulum, so increasing bladder capacity and hopefully thereby lowering bladder pressure.

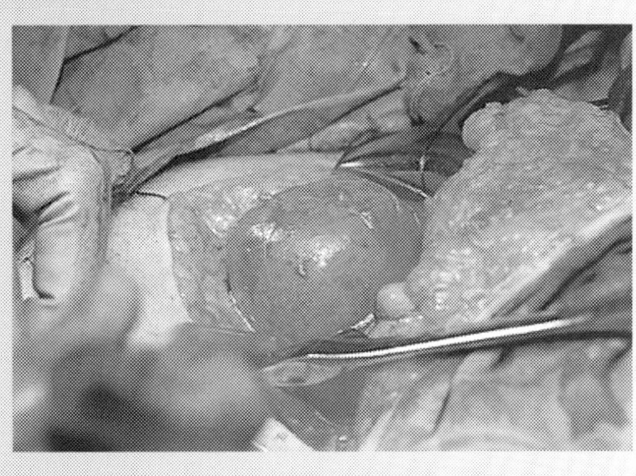

medication or clam cystoplasty has failed to make them dry, then an additional procedure may be necessary to increase urethral resistance to a level where they are dry. This can take the form of a periurethral sling or implantation of an artificial urinary sphincter. A periurethral sling can be fashioned from a strip of rectus fascia or commercially available materials may be used. The sling angulates the urethra, rather in the way that one kinks a garden hose to stop the flow of water. The artifical urinary sphincter (*Fig. 6.5*) essentially consists of two balloons connected, via fine-bore plastic tubing, by a control pump which is located in the scrotum or labia majora (*Fig. 6.6*). One of the balloons is configured as a cuff (which is placed around the urethra) and the other is a large reservoir (usually placed deep to one of the rectus muscles). The pressure head normally directs fluid from the reservoir to the cuff, maintaining the cuff in an inflated state, so occluding the urethra and maintaining continence. When the patient wishes to empty their bladder, they squeeze the pump once or twice and this forces fluid out of the cuff into the reservoir balloon. The cuff deflates, they empty their bladder (spontaneously or by ISC) and then

Fig. 6.5:
An AMS800 artificial urinary sphincter.

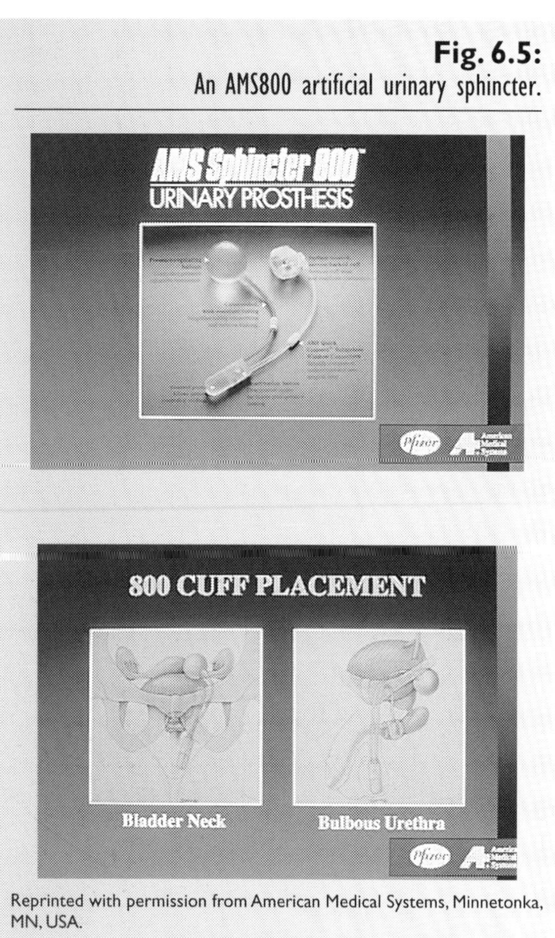

Reprinted with permission from American Medical Systems, Minnetonka, MN, USA.

Fig. 6.6:
Diagrammatic representation of the AMS800 artificial urinary sphincter. It essentially consists of two balloons connected, via fine bore plastic tubing, to a control pump which is located in the scrotum or labia majora.

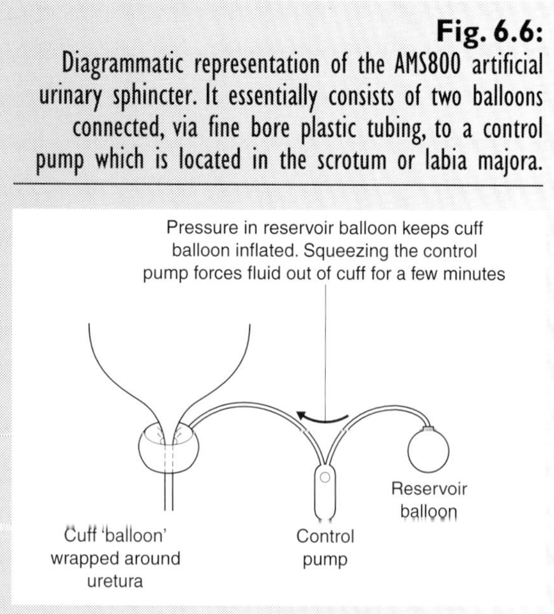

over the course of the next few minutes the cuff slowly reinflates, so again maintaining continence. The AMS800 is a highly refined and mechanically very simple device (which has taken years of painstaking development). It can be a very effective way of achieving continence. As with any foreign material implanted into the body, one potential complication is device infection, which almost always necessitates removal and as with any mechanical device it has a finite lifespan (though this may be many years).

An alternative procedure for lowering bladder pressure in combined detrusor hyperreflexia and DESD (e.g. in men with spinal cord injuries) is to divide the posterior roots (posterior rhizotomy) from the bladder (the sensory nerves) and to implant a sacral anterior root stimulator (SARS). Division of the posterior roots interrupts the sacral reflex arc to the bladder (effectively a lower motor neuron lesion) creating an atonic (flaccid) bladder and sphincter (continued function of the bladder neck maintains continence). The anterior root stimulator is then switched on when the patient wishes to void (a small external transducer is applied over an internal transducer which has been buried under the skin, and activation of the external transducer activates bladder emptying). Stimulation of the sacral anterior roots (the motor supply to the bladder) causes a bladder contraction and the bladder empties. Division of the posterior roots and implantation of a SARS is a complex neurosurgical procedure, and when a patient has some degree of preservation of sensation in the distribution of the sacral posterior roots they may be reluctant to lose this by posterior rhizotomy. However, when the procedure works, it can be a very good way of lowering bladder pressures, maintaining continence and protecting the kidneys, and at achieving efficient bladder emptying.

One of the most important factors in treating and preventing urinary tract infection in patients with neuropathic bladders is to achieve efficient bladder emptying. In this respect ISC, external sphincterotomy or a SARS can all be very effective. It is worth emphasizing that a patient who is performing ISC who develops a urinary infection should catheterize **more** frequently, rather than less frequently – to improve bladder emptying and to prevent a pool of stagnant, infected urine from remaining in the bladder. It is a commonly held misconception that ISC is the **cause** of recurrent infections, but as long as the patient follows basic rules of hygiene, it is unusual for them to infect themselves. I have a patient (a farmer) who catheterizes himself on his tractor while working in his fields and since increasing the frequency of ISC his recurrent UTIs have stopped! Persistent or recurrent infections in a patient with a neuropathic bladder (and indeed in a neurologically normal individual) is an indication for upper tract imaging (a plain abdominal X-ray and renal ultrasound), looking specifically for renal calculi (particularly staghorn stones – a classic cause of recurrent urinary tract infection).

Key points

- Bladder and sphincter contraction have a reciprocal relationship, such that when the bladder is relaxed the sphincter is contracted (during bladder filling) and continence is maintained. Conversely, when the bladder contracts, the sphincter relaxes (during micturition) for a sufficient time to allow complete bladder emptying to occur.
- Disturbance of this normal relationship in certain types of neurologic conditions (such as spinal cord injury or spina bifida) is called detrusor-sphincter dyssynergia and this can cause a profound degree of bladder outlet obstruction.
- The neuropathic bladder may have contractile dysfunction, intermediate dysfunction or be acontractile. Contractile and intermediate type bladders can cause high bladder and intrarenal pressures and are thus potentially 'dangerous' bladders.
- Whenever you see a patient with a neuropathic bladder, you should think 'how good is this patient's bladder at emptying?' and 'what is their bladder pressure?'.
- Complex urodynamic tests are only required if the patient has a persistent problem, in terms of continence or renal function, after simple measures designed to improve bladder emptying have been tried and failed.

Cases

1. A 40-year-old man presents with painful urinary retention. His prostate is small and benign, and he reports a preceding history of loss of orgasms, and a burning sensation in his penis and scrotum over the last 4 weeks.
   (a) What are the key points in examination?
   (b) Which one single further investigation should you obtain?

2. A paraplegic male patient with an acontractile bladder and normal hand function has been performing ISC for 2 years with no problems. However, over the last 6 months he has had 6 UTIs.
   (a) Which investigations would you order?
   (b) If these are normal, what advice would you give him?

3. A 30-year-old T6 paraplegic woman has been performing ISC for 2 years since her accident, but continues to leak urine in-between catheterizing herself. She has been on full doses of anticholinergic drugs with no improvement. She does not want a long-term suprapubic catheter. What investigation would be helpful in determining subsequent management and what is her next treatment option?

Answers

1. (a) A young man with urinary retention has a neurological cause for this until proven otherwise. His history of seemingly odd sensations in the genitalia and sexual dysfunction are highly suggestive of a neurological basis for retention. Neurological examination is crucial, and you should specifically test for power and reflexes in the legs, sensation around the perianal and in particular pericoccygeal region and determine whether the patient has a positive bulbocavernosus reflex. If this is absent, he almost certainly has a cord lesion, though given his symptoms a positive BCR should not be taken as evidence that there is nothing wrong with him.
   (b) He should have an MRI scan of his spinal cord and cauda equina.

2. (a) He should have a KUB (kidneys, ureters, bladder) X-ray and renal and bladder ultrasound to exclude renal tract stones and assess bladder emptying. Patients with neurological disease affecting bladder function are at high risk for development of kidney and bladder stones, and these often present not with pain, but with a history of recurrent UTIs or evidence of increased autonomic dysreflexia (bladder spasms – causing leakage of urine, headaches, and increased leg spasms).
   (b) You should ask him how many times a day he is catheterizing himself and if this is only 3 or 4 times, suggest that he increase the frequency of ISC to 6 or 7 times a day, and possibly once in the middle of the night.

3. She should undergo urodynamic investigation which will probably show that she has a high-pressure bladder, which is filling up to a certain (low) volume and the detrusor pressures are then overcoming her urethral pressures. She has essentially failed medical therapy (ISC and full-dose anticholinergic medication). Surgical options include augmentation of her bladder with bowel, which will increase her capacity and thereby lower her detrusor pressure. This in itself may be enough for her urethral sphincter to be able to keep her dry. Her subsequent bladder pressures may be so low that she may not be able to pass any urine at all, but as long as she is happy to do ISC and can do this effectively (i.e. achieve good bladder emptying) this is not a problem. An alternative procedure is division of her posterior sacral roots (which effectively will render her bladder areflexic – a lower motor neuron type bladder), followed by implantation of a sacral anterior root stimulator, which is activated each time her bladder is full and she wishes to void. This is a major neurosurgical procedure.

References

Kaplan A.S., Chancellor M.B., Blaivas J.G. Bladder and sphincter behaviour in patients with spinal cord lesions. *J Urol* 1996; **146**: 113–117.

Lapides J., Diokno A.C., Silber S.J., Lowe B.S. Clean intermittent self-catheterization in the treatment of urinary tract disease. *J Urol* 1972; **107**: 458.

Mundy A.R. The neuropathic bladder. Introduction and patient selection for surgery. In: *Controversises and Innovations in Urological Surgery*. Eds Gingell C, Abrams P. Springer-Verlag, Berlin. 1988, pp. 203–210.

CHAPTER 7

Adult urological infection

Introduction

Infection of the urinary tract is the most common bacterial infection of humans of all ages and a huge problem throughout the world. Not only in terms of its morbidity and occasional mortality, but also in terms of the cost of resources required to treat it. It affects women much more than men and it has been estimated that 50% of women will suffer one or more symptomatic urinary tract infections in her lifetime. The features of urinary tract infection (UTI) are listed in *Table 7.1*. *Figure 7.1* demonstrates the spectrum of urinary tract infections.

A quarter of patients who experience a UTI go on to get recurrent infections. Although acute bacterial infection is the commonest problem in the West, the chronic infections of tuberculosis and schistosomiasis are still common in other parts of the world.

The urinary tract is normally sterile above the distal urethra. This is due to several reasons. The dilution of bacteria by the flow of urine. The secretion of immunoglobulin A (IgA) by the mucosa and the protective capability of the urothelium itself. In the case of bacteria causing ascending infection, adherence to uroepithelial cells is a key factor in determining virulence. Bacterial adhesins produced by pili on the bacterial surface interact with specific receptors on the urothelial surface. This mechanism is important in pathogenesis and a good example of this is the *P. fimbriae* possessed by *E. coli*. Factors predisposing to UTI are listed in *Table 7.2*.

Fig. 7.1:
The spectrum of urinary tract infections.

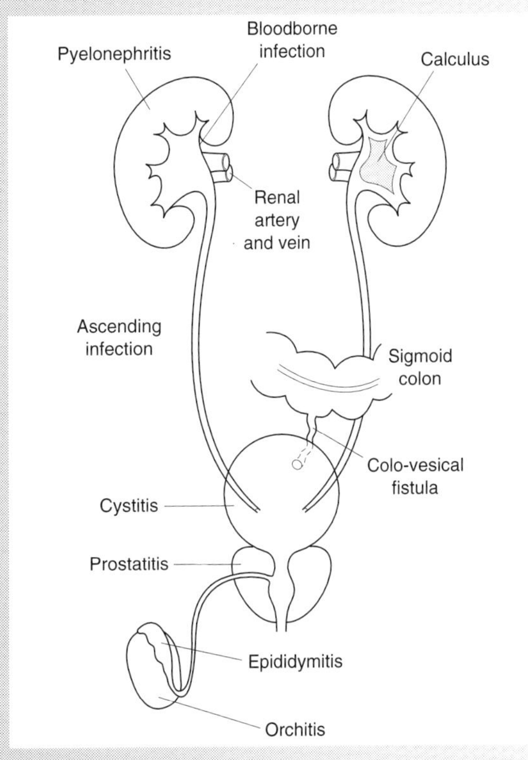

Redrawn from *Essential Urology 1st Edn.*, Bullock *et al.*, Fig. 8.1, 1989, by permission of the publisher Churchill Livingstone.

Table 7.1:
Features of UTI

Experienced by 1 in 5 women
25% of those affected have recurrent infections
Men get it but much less commonly due to increased urethral length
Ascending infection causes pyelonephritis with loin pain, fever and malaise

Bacteria enter the bladder through the bloodstream or the urethra when these defence mechanisms break down. In the latter case ascending infection will carry them up to the kidneys where pyelonephritis can develop with loin pain, fever and malaise.

The common pathogens are listed in *Table 7.3*.

Table 7.2:
Factors predisposing to infection

Retained urine due to obstruction or congenital dilatation
Catheters, ureteric stents or other foreign bodies
Conditions that lead to immunosuppression: diabetes, organ transplants, chemotherapy
Fistulae between the bladder and bowel e.g. diverticular disease

Table 7.3:
The commonest bacterial causes of UTI

Escherichia coli
Streptococcus faecalis (now *Enterococcus*)
Proteus mirabilis
Klebsiella sp.
Pseudomonas aeruginosa
Staphylococcus epidermidis

Upper urinary tract infections

These may be acute or chronic infections. Most are due to ascending infection and for this reason 75% are associated with lower urinary tract symptoms.

Acute pyelonephritis

Pathology

This is the most common upper urinary tact infection which causes acute inflammation of the renal pelvis, calyces and renal parenchyma. It is usually due to ascending infection with bacteria entering the kidney via the ureter, renal pelvis and collecting ducts.

Clinical features

The two classic symptoms of renal infection are pyrexia and loin pain. Rigors are not uncommon due to the release of bacteria into the bloodstream and septicaemia may occur, especially if infection is associated with obstruction. In this case the patient will be very sick with hypotension, poor peripheral perfusion and circulatory collapse.

Investigations and diagnosis

The most important investigation is examination of the urine for leucocytes, bacteria and casts. Blood cultures should be taken from all patients with pyrexia or a clinical suspicion of septicaemia.

A plain abdominal X-ray may show a calculus and there may be a soft-tissue mass with absence of the psoas shadow on the affected side. Ultrasound will detect hydronephrosis from obstruction. An IVU may show enlargement of the infected kidney with poor concentration of contrast medium in acute pyelonephritis but a CT urogram will usually give much better information about the kidney.

Treatment

Antibiotic therapy is the mainstay of treatment for uncomplicated acute pyelonephritis. The treatment should be tailored to the patients needs and this depends on the type of infection present, and its severity. Often intravenous antibiotics are required in the initial stages and as the infection comes under control these can be changed to oral antibiotics. It is often wise to continue these for at least 2 weeks to try and prevent relapse. The urine should then be monitored for infection after stopping the antibiotics to detect recurrent or relapsing infection.

In the severely ill and septicaemia patient, emergency resuscitation may be required to treat circulatory collapse. Intravenous antibiotics (gentamycin and ampicillin is a good combination) should be given after blood cultures have been taken.

Complications

The two main complications of acute pyelonephritis are pyonephrosis and perinephric abscess (*Fig. 7.2*). Pyonephrosis is the result of infection within an obstructed kidney. The obstruction may be chronic or acute. Prompt drainage under antibiotic cover is vital to prevent irreversible renal damage. This is best achieved by percutaneous nephrostomy performed under local anaesthetic. Sometimes the pus from the kidney is too thick to drain down the small cannulae that are inserted in this way so that formal surgical drainage and operative placement

Fig. 7.2:
Acute renal infections.

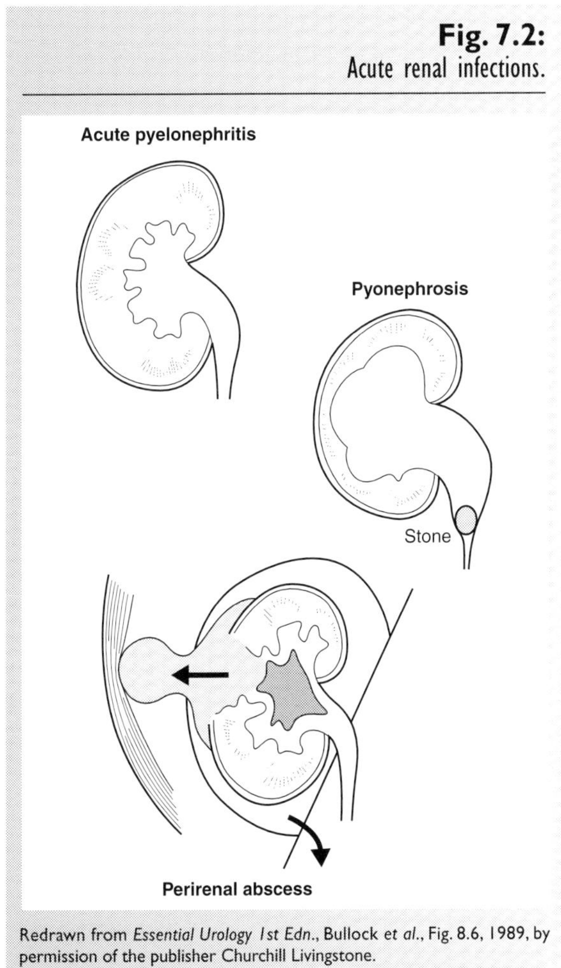

Redrawn from *Essential Urology 1st Edn.*, Bullock *et al.*, Fig. 8.6, 1989, by permission of the publisher Churchill Livingstone.

Fig. 7.3:
Calcification on a ureteric stent.

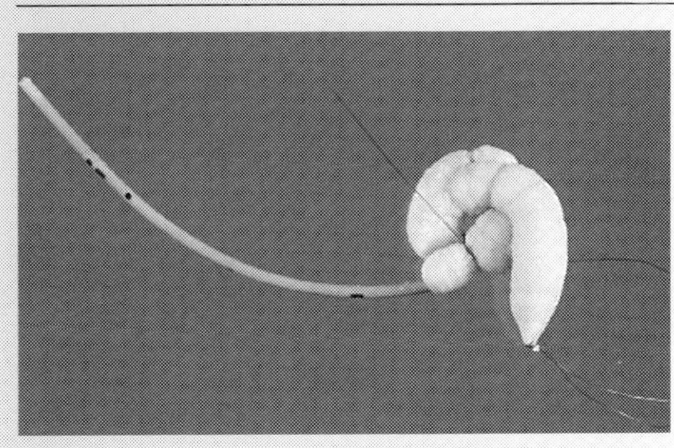

of a large nephrostomy tube may be necessary. Occasionally, the collecting system can be drained from below with a ureteric catheter (J stent) passed from the bladder at cystoscopy. If this is placed in patients with stone disease it should be removed as soon as possible to prevent further stone formation around the stent (*Fig. 7.3*). If the renal function is poor and does not improve with drainage, it is best to perform a nephrectomy.

A perinephric abscess can result from acute pyelonephritis. Initially, the infection is confined by Gerota's fascia but may then rupture through this to reach adjacent organs such as the psoas muscle or the bowel or even the skin through the lumbar triangle.

Surgical drainage under antibiotic cover is required. The precipitating cause should be dealt with in a kidney, which functions well, but, if function in the affected kidney is very poor, nephrectomy is the treatment of choice.

Chronic pyelonephritis

Pathology

Chronic pyelonephritis can be obstructive or non-obstructive in nature. Both give rise to recurrent infection and renal scarring (*Fig. 7.4*). In the non-obstructive situation the cause may be due to vesico-ureteric reflux (*Fig. 7.5*) and infection in childhood or may develop in adult life as a result of persistent bacteriuria between repeated episodes of acute pyelonephritis.

Clinical features

Patients may present either with recurrent symptomatic UTIs or the infection may be subclinical with bacteriuria detected only on routine urine screening.

Occasionally, the disease presents at an advanced stage when chronic renal failure has occurred. In this situation the patient will present with all the symptoms of renal failure (see Chapter 12).

Investigations and diagnosis

The diagnosis can be established by the finding of infection in the urine and cortical scarring which

Fig. 7.4:
Cortical scarring associated with chronic pyelonephritis.

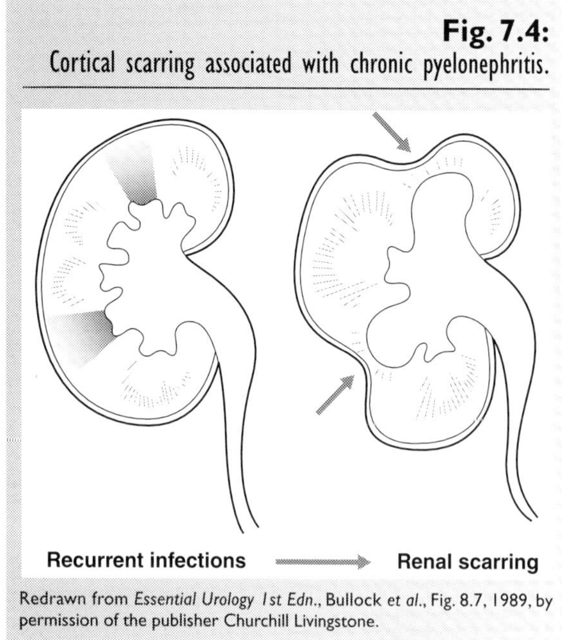

Redrawn from *Essential Urology 1st Edn.*, Bullock *et al.*, Fig. 8.7, 1989, by permission of the publisher Churchill Livingstone.

Fig. 7.5:
Micturating cystogram showing reflux in a Duplex system.

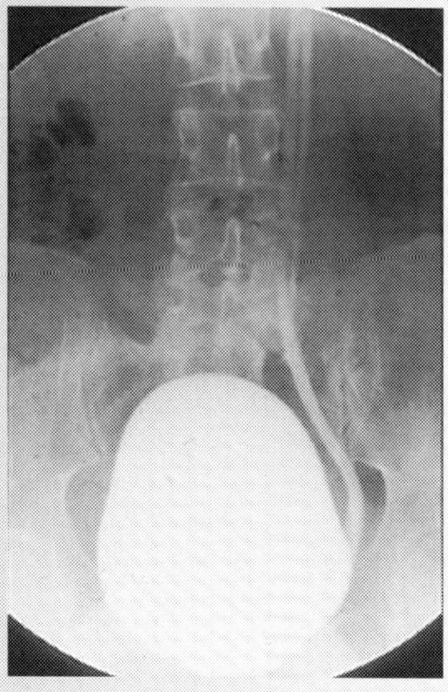

overlies a deformed calyx on the ultrasound, IVU or CT scan. In chronic renal failure, the kidneys may appear small and scarred on ultrasound imaging, and show diminished function on renography.

Treatment

Any predisposing cause for persistent infection should be dealt with as appropriate. Treatment is then aimed at eliminating infection and preventing further renal damage. Symptomatic infections should be treated with an appropriate antibiotic and long-term low-dose antibiotics should be considered.

Nephrectomy may occasionally be required for a severely diseased kidney or for severe symptoms, provided the contralateral kidney is normal. This may be performed by open or laparoscopic approach. If scarring and damage are confined to one pole of the kidney, a partial nephrectomy can be performed to preserve as many functioning nephrons as possible.

Complications

Chronic pyelonephritis may cause serious renal damage and remains a significant cause of end-stage renal failure accounting for 15% of adult cases and 30% of childhood cases. Renal replacement therapy in the form of dialysis or transplantation will be necessary for patients with end-stage renal failure.

Lower urinary tract infections

Acute bacterial cystitis

In some patients, the urine may contain bacteria nearly all the time whilst, in others, recurrent bouts of infection occur with periods of sterile urine in between. Symptoms vary considerably, from minor frequency to recurrent episodes of severe acute cystitis.

Pathology

This is usually the result of ascending infection from the perineum. It is much more common in women, with over half of all women experiencing at least one attack during their lifetime. The reasons for this higher incidence in women than men is due to the shorter length of the female urethra;

and its position which is readily contaminated with faecal organisms. In postmenopausal women, atrophic vaginitis is a predisposing factor for recurrent urinary tract infections due to a decrease in resistance to ascending infection.

In men and children, infection is more likely to be associated with some abnormality of the urinary tract.

Clinical features

The clinical features of urinary tract infection are frequency and urgency of micturition with dysuria. There may be suprapubic pain between voiding and there may be associated haematuria. Occasionally fever and rigors may be present from associated bacteraemia. There may be spread to the kidneys with associated loin pain.

Examination is usually unremarkable, although the temperature may be elevated and there may be suprapubic tenderness. Occasionally, there are signs related to upper tract involvement or an underlying abnormality predisposing to the infection.

Investigations and diagnosis

The dipstick urinalysis is a useful diagnostic tool. The leucocyte esterase test detects pus cells and the nitrate reductase test detects bacteria that reduce nitrate to nitrite. A mid-stream urine (MSU) for microscopy, culture and sensitivity to antibiotics confirms a UTI which is usually present with $>10^5$ bacterial forming colonies ml^{-1}. Interstitial cystitis and bladder cancer both present as UTIs in unusual circumstances and must not be forgotten as a differential diagnosis.

Further investigations are indicated if there are three repeated episodes of cystitis in women but a single episode in men.

Renal function should be checked by measuring the plasma creatinine and electrolytes of all patients that need investigating. An ultrasound scan of the renal tract is relatively non-invasive, in the majority of patients this will be all that is needed. A renal ultrasound shows the thickness of the renal cortex and the presence of calculi, scarring or obstruction. A bladder scan will exclude residual urine and stones. If the USS scan and clinical features together raise the possibility of ureteric reflux, the patient will need to have a micturating cystogram. Patients with very frequent infections and very intrusive symptoms or haematuria will warrant a referral for cystoscopy to examine the bladder, and indeed may benefit from urethral dilatation done at the same time (*Table 7.4*).

Treatment

Simple measures that help include increased fluid intake and alkalinizing agents such as sodium bicarbonate or potassium citrate if the urine pH is less than 6. A suitable antibiotic should be started immediately and given for a 5-day period; this can be changed, if necessary, on the basis of antibiotic sensitivity tests.

If the initial course of antibiotics produces resolution of symptoms, the MSU should be repeated at 2 weeks and again at 3 months to ensure that infection has been eradicated.

All women with recurrent UTIs should be given advice about hygiene, bladder emptying, and the quantity and nature of their fluid intake (*Table 7.5*). Drinks containing caffeine and alcohol are definitely associated with frequency and urgency, and may be associated with more frequent infections. They should therefore be limited. Cranberry juice has been used for decades in the USA as a folk remedy for UTI. While it seems to have no direct antibacterial effect there is evidence to suggest that cranberry juice is effective in interfering with the bacterial adherence to uroepithelium which would render bacteria susceptible to elimination by flushing.

Table 7.4:
Investigations for UTI

Serum creatinine and electrolytes
X-ray of kidneys, ureters and bladder (KUB)
Renal ultrasound (USS) for stones, scarring
Bladder USS for residual volume combined with uroflowmetry
Micturating cystourethrogram if renal scarring is present on USS

Table 7.5:
Preventing UTIs in women

Wear cotton underwear
Always wipe from front to back after micturition or defecation
Drink plenty of fluid (approximately half a pint every 2 hours) but limit caffeine-containing drinks (coffee, tea) and alcohol. Try cranberry juice
Empty the bladder after intercourse
Wash the genital area regularly, but avoid bubble baths, personal deodorants and talcum powder
Take sodium bicarbonate or potassium citrate to reduce urinary acidity
Pass urine regularly, and make sure the bladder is completely emptied. Practise 'double micturition'

There is occasionally a role for long-term antibiotics, but these should be used only for those with very frequent infections and/or very intrusive symptoms.

There is no clear evidence of benefit from rotating through different antibiotics. Instead, a regular night-time dose of trimethroprim (or other appropriate antibiotic acceptable to the patient) should be given for 3–6 months and then discontinued while symptoms are monitored.

Treatment of atrophic vaginitis in post-menopausal women with hormone replacement therapy can certainly lead to a lessening of frequency and dysuria.

In men with evidence of prostatic enlargement and outflow obstruction, surgery to the bladder neck or prostate may be necessary.

Chronic cystitis

Pathology

Chronic inflammation in the bladder may be due to recurrent bacterial infections, but more often is due to other causes, which are listed in *Table 7.6*.

Histologically, the chronically inflamed bladder may show cystic changes or squamous metaplasia. Squamous cell carcinoma of the bladder can occur from chronic irritation, in particular in patients with schistosomiasis, long-term catheters or calculi.

Table 7.6:
Causes of chronic cystitis

Long-term catheter
Untreated bladder stones
Toxic drugs and chemicals e.g. cyclophosphamide
Radiotherapy
Viruses e.g. adenoviruses
Parasitic infections e.g. schistosomiasis
Interstitial cystitis
Colovesical fistula

Interstitial cystitis has an obscure aetiology and is characterized by an inflammatory infiltrate with mast cells in the submucosa, which may subsequently lead to fibrosis.

Clinical features

These are the same as the acute infections but tend to be chronic in nature with urgency frequency both day and night. Often there is suprapubic or perineal pain that may be relieved for a short time by micturition, then recur again after a short period of time. Pneumaturia indicates a colovesical fistula.

Investigations and diagnosis

Urine testing including cytology is essential and investigation of the urinary tract with a plain film and ultrasound is useful to identify any underlying problems. Cystoscopy and urethral dilatation helps a proportion of women and allows examination and biopsy of the bladder to exclude malignancy and help to clarify the diagnosis. Barium enema may demonstrate colovesical fistula.

Treatment

Any underlying cause should be treated where possible. Interstitial cystitis is notoriously difficult to treat. Various bladder instillations may help including dimethylsulphoxide and cystistat. Cystoscopy and short or long bladder distension are often effective on a temporary basis, and can be repeated. Rarely cystoplasty to enlarge the bladder, or even a total cystectomy and bladder reconstruction or urinary diversion or excision of colovesical fistula may be necessary.

Complications

Squamous bladder cancer may develop in areas of squamous metaplasia in longstanding inflammation.

Prostatitis

Pathology

Prostatitis may be due to acute or chronic bacterial infection and non-bacterial prostatitis can also occur in the absence of bacterial growth, and it has been suggested that chronic pelvic pain syndrome would be a more appropriate term for this group of patients without demonstrable infection. Demonstrations of bacteria in the post-prostatic massage of urine or expressed prostatic secretions when the midstream urine shows no growth is highly diagnostic of bacterial prostatitis. *Escherichia coli* or *Klebsiella* and *Proteus* are the species that most often cause bacterial prostatitis. *Pseudomonas* and *Enterococcus* are less common.

Clinical features

Acute bacterial prostatitis is often associated with generalized malaise and fever associated with symptoms localized to the prostate and acute cystitis. It is seen in men of all ages and typically is associated with pain in the perineum and suprapubic areas associated with frequency and urgency of micturition. Abdominal examination is normally unremarkable but the characteristic feature is a very tender prostate on rectal examination. Occasionally a fluctuant abscess may be palpable within the prostate.

Investigations and diagnosis

Expressed prostatic secretions from prostatic massage may reveal the presence of leucocytes or bacteria. Ultrasound scan of the kidneys and bladder reveals any gross abnormality of the urinary tract that will predispose to infection. Transrectal ultrasound scanning gives a good view of the prostate and will show any abnormal areas or the presence of a prostatic abscess. Serum prostatic specific antigen (PSA) levels in the blood are often raised in prostatitis and should be interpreted with caution. Cystoscopy and biopsy of any abnormal areas in the prostatic urethra or bladder will exclude bladder carcinoma in situ, which has been known to masquerade as prostatitis.

Treatment

Bacterial prostatitis or epididymitis responds well to antimicrobial drugs. It is necessary to treat the patients over a prolonged period to prevent the development of chronic bacterial prostatitis for at least 6 weeks.

Chronic bacterial prostatitis is one of the most common causes of relapsing urinary tract infection in men and in the past has been difficult to treat, although the fluoroquinolone antibiotics have been shown to be safe and effective in treatment of this condition (e.g. ciprofloxacin).

Non-bacterial prostatitis is more common than bacterial prostatitis, although the aetiology is unknown and the treatment often empirical and of variable effectiveness. Chlamydia remains a possible aetiological agent although the evidence for its role is far from definite. A trial of tetracycline or one of its derivatives, associated with α-adrenergic blocking agents are sometimes of help, especially in patients with perineal pain from the prostate, as the prostate is known to be rich in α-adrenergic receptors, and symptoms may be relieved by these drugs.

Complications

Prostatic abscess can develop which is best drained transurethrally rather than rectally to avoid the possibility of creating a prostato-rectal fistula. Chronic pain is a feature of chronic prostatitis and this may be exacerbated by concern as to likelihood of prostatic carcinoma as a diagnosis.

Epididymitis and orchitis

Pathology

Infection may involve the epididymis alone (epididymitis), the testis alone (orchitis) or both organs (epididymo-orchitis). Epididymitis is much more common than orchitis but most patients with clinical evidence of epididymitis usually have some testicular involvement. Although the epididymis is the predominant site of pathology the majority of cases of epididymitis have an infectious aetiology, and the initial infection arises in the urethra, prostate or bladder. Infection can come from the blood stream, from direct extension along the vas deferens itself or through associated lymphatic channels to colonize and infect the epididymis.

Clinical features

The onset of epididymo-orchitis is often sudden and in younger patients difficult to differentiate from testicular torsion. There is pain and swelling of the scrotum. Symptoms of UTI may be present, and if the infection is severe there may be systemic symptoms with fever and rigors. There may be a history of urethral discharge or sexual disease or instrumentation. In many cases no cause is identified.

The epididymis and testis are swollen and it may be impossible to distinguish between them. A secondary hydrocele may be present.

Investigations and diagnosis

In boys and young men the main differential diagnosis of epididymitis (and orchitis) is torsion of the testis which requires emergency surgery. Torsion of the testis is most common between 12 and 18 years and rare under the age of 2.

Microscopic examination of the urine and/or urethral discharge may be helpful in differentiating epididymitis from torsion since pyuria or bacteriuria is frequently present in epididymitis but is not found with torsion. Doppler ultrasonography has been used to evaluate blood flow to the affected scrotum; epididymitis is associated with increased blood flow whereas torsion results in decreased blood flow. But this does not invariably correlate with surgical findings, and if there is any doubt about the diagnosis the testicle should be explored, for leaving an undiagnosed torsion not only destroys one testicle but also leaves the other at risk from subsequent torsion as the abnormality is bilateral.

Treatment

In addition to symptomatic treatment such as bed rest, scrotal elevation and analgesia, antibiotics should always be given as the majority of cases have a microbial aetiology. Since the routine use of antibiotics in these patients the incidence of subsequent abscess formation and testicular infarction has decreased. The commonest organisms are *E. coli* and *Chlamydia*. For the former, ciprofloxacin is a good choice, while for the latter, doxycycline is effective. Treatment is often necessary for up to 6 weeks to prevent relapse.

Complications

The main complications are abscess formation and testicular infarction. Any inflammation which also involves the testis may affect fertility. This will not be evident if only one testis is involved but may be if both are affected.

Viral orchitis

Pathology

Mumps virus is the most frequent aetiological agent of orchitis, although it can complicate other viral illnesses. Mumps orchitis usually appears 4–6 days after the onset of parotitis, although it rarely occurs in the absence of clinical parotitis.

It occurs in 20% of men over puberty that contract mumps. It is unilateral in 80% of cases and subsides in 7–10 days.

Clinical features

Clinical manifestations of orchitis are high fever and swollen, painful testicles, which are very tender and appear somewhat soft. The effect on the semen depends on the presence of testicular atrophy and whether the orchitis is unilateral or bilateral.

Investigations and diagnosis

Parotitis is usually present and the diagnosis is confirmed on a rising titre of anti-mumps antibody. If torsion cannot be excluded the testis must be explored.

Treatment

The orchitis will resolve on its own, but symptomatic treatment in the form of bed rest, scrotal support and analgesia will help.

Complications
Testicular atrophy occurs in one out of every two or three men with viral orchitis. Fertility may be impaired if the orchitis is bilateral as with other causes of orchitis.

Balanitis

Pathology
Balanitis is inflammation of the foreskin, but this often affects the glans penis when the condition is known as balanoposthitis. These conditions are common in men with a long, tight prepuce whose hygiene is poor and it is also common in diabetic men.

Clinical features
There may be swelling or redness of the foreskin. If the foreskin is tight and pale with pallor extending onto the glans the condition is known as balanitis xerotica obliterans which is the genital manifestation of the skin condition lichen sclerosis et atrophicus; initial patchy erythema progresses to atrophy with a white appearance, meatal stenosis and phimosis.

Investigations and diagnosis
The blood sugar should be checked to exclude diabetes, the condition is diagnosed from the clinical appearance.

Treatment
Local saline bathing is always advised and is sufficient in mild to moderate cases and when no cause is found. Antibiotics may be appropriate, hydrocortisone cream 1% is useful in more severe cases of BXO. If a tight phimosis remains after treatment then circumcision should be offered.

Complications
The two main complications of balanitis are phimosis and meatal stenosis.

Unusual infections

Tuberculosis of the urinary tract

Pathology
Although uncommon in the UK it is still seen, and on a worldwide basis is common. The organism is usually *Mycobacterium tuberculosis* and renal infection occurs through haematogeneous spread, although less than 5% of patients with pulmonary TB go on to develop genitourinary tuberculosis, probably because most of the microscopic miliary tubercles that reach the renal cortex resolve. If they do not the first sign of abnormality may be frequency and haematuria from small lesions developing in the papilla and this may extend deeper into the cortex to form an abscess and often calcifies. The calyces may narrow causing obstruction and if untreated can lead to destruction of the kidney.

Clinical features
The usual presenting features are lower urinary tract symptoms, often with haematuria. Loin pain may be related to obstruction to the kidneys, and tuberculosis in the genital area can result in a thickened enlarged epididymis. Progressive involvement of the ureter can lead to thickening and stricture formation in the ureter and tuberculous cystitis leads to fibrosis and contracture of the bladder with symptoms of frequency and urgency often with haematuria. Biopsy may reveal acid-fast bacilli and tubercles. MSU typically shows sterile pyuria.

Treatment
Diagnosis is by early morning urine samples (EMUs) looking for acid-fast bacilli with the Ziehl-Neelsen stain. Ultrasound may show obstruction and IVU may reveal obstruction and ureteric strictures.

A full course of anti-tuberculous treatment is instigated and the patients are usually managed jointly with chest physicians or infectious disease specialists. Occasionally nephrectomy may be necessary, although auto-nephrectomy from the consequences of the disease is sometimes seen.

Complications

Ureteric strictures may require stents. Surgery to correct a contracted bladder by cystoplasty and bowel augmentation is sometimes helpful (*Fig. 7.6*).

Schistosomiasis (Bilharzia)

Pathology

Schistosomiasis is a huge problem world wide, and one of the major causes of squamous cell carcinoma of the bladder due to irritation by the ova in the wall of the bladder. It is caused by the adult trematode fluke *Schistosoma haematobium* (*Table 7.7*). They are flat worms with life cycles that spend one stage in molluscs and one stage in vertebrates (*Fig. 7.7*).

Table 7.7:
Types of schistosoma

Schistosoma haematobium	Africa, Caribbean, Brazil
Schistosoma mansoni	Africa, Caribbean, Brazil
Schistosoma japonicum	Far East

The adult flukes are 5 mm in length and are attached by a sucker to the inside of human veins. The name is derived from the Greek split (schisto) body (soma) due to the fact that the male enfolds the female in a long split down his body. Bilharz, a German pathologist working in Egypt, discovered the

Fig. 7.6:
Changes seen in tuberculosis of the urinary tract.

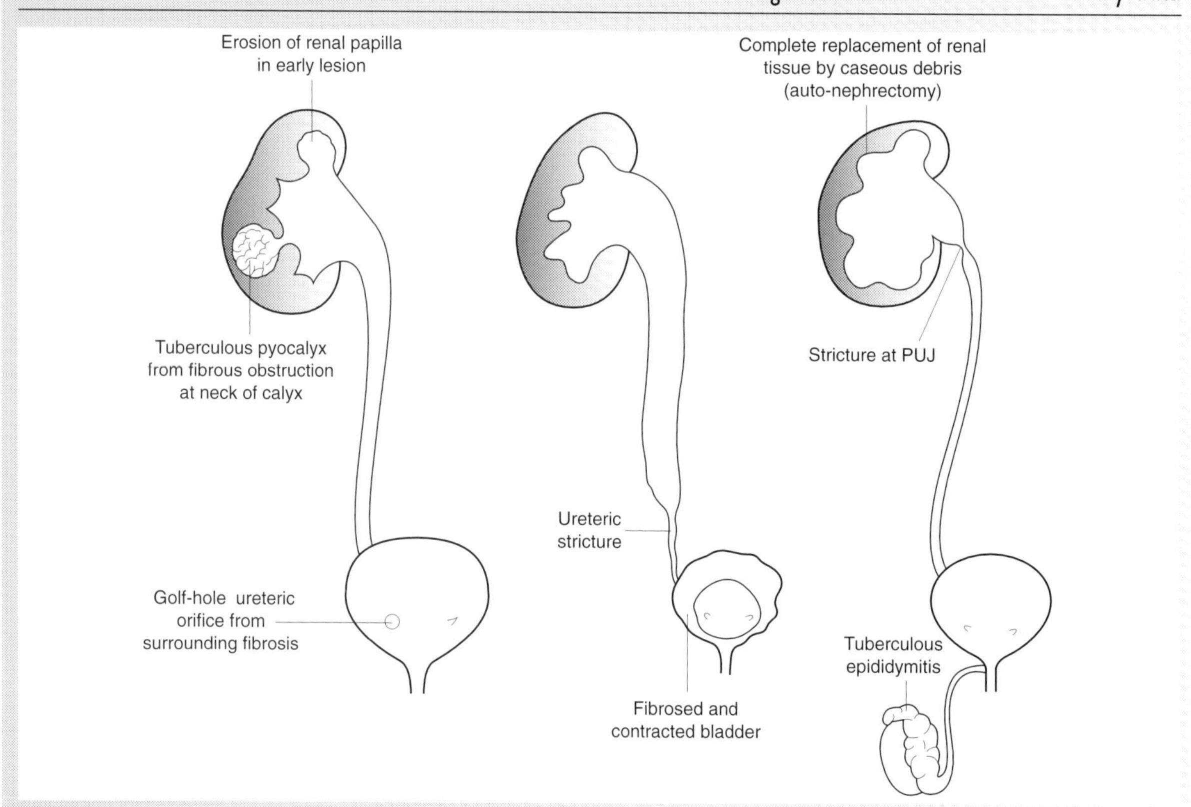

Redrawn from *Essential Urology 1st Edn.*, Bullock *et al.*, Fig. 8.8, 1989, by permission of the publisher Churchill Livingstone.

Fig. 7.7:
The life cycle of schistosomiasis.

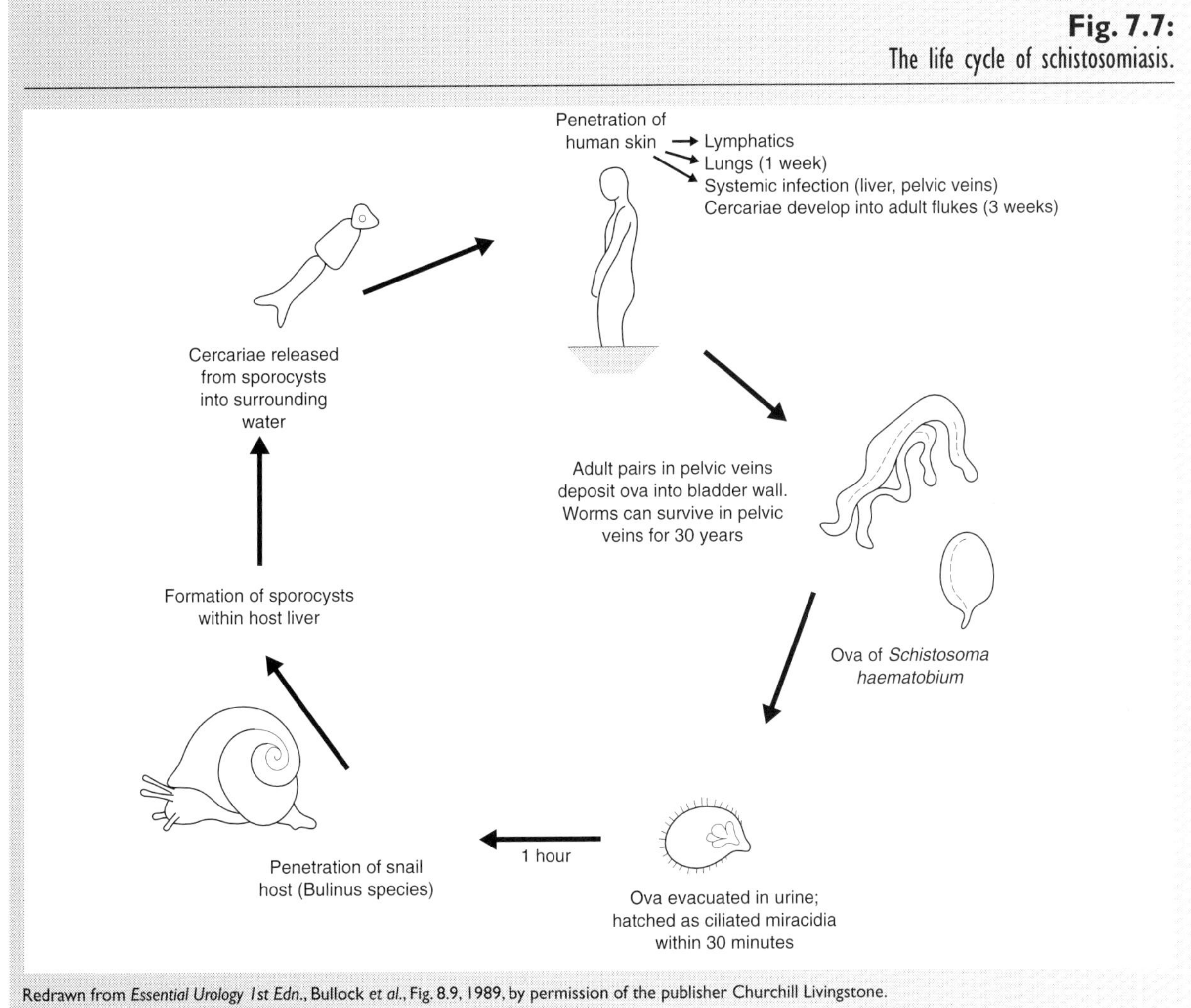

Redrawn from *Essential Urology 1st Edn.*, Bullock *et al.*, Fig. 8.9, 1989, by permission of the publisher Churchill Livingstone.

disease and he found these worms in the portal veins of children who had died with portal hypertension. The disease is still called Bilharzia for this reason.

Clinical

The classic means of developing the disease is swimming in infected water, and it is seen in people returning to the UK after spending time swimming in infected areas. It is common for the flukes to live in the veins around the bladder and portal veins although they can go anywhere and live and dead eggs can work their way submucosally where they cause haematuria and lower urinary tract symptoms. Later on fibrosis may lead to a much reduced bladder capacity.

Investigation

The diagnosis is made by identification of schistosomal eggs in the urine or bladder biopsies. An enzyme linked immunosorbent assay is also available. The cystoscopic appearance is of sand-like particles within the bladder.

Treatment

This is with praziquantel on a single day in 2 or 3 doses. While this is effective for treatment of tourists who have picked it up abroad, the local population who live in infested areas will not be rid of it until the habitat or their life style changes.

Complications

These are related to the fibrosis around the ova and the irritation caused by the ova. In the first case, ureteric obstruction and hydronephrosis can develop, in the second case it is the chronic irritation of the ova in the bladder that leads to the development of squamous cell cancer of the bladder.

Xanthogranulomatous pyelonephritis

This is the result of a granulomatous reaction within the kidney to chronic infection and is usually related to longstanding renal stones and obstruction. Although it may occur in diabetics and usually only involves one kidney.

Pathology

The granulomatous response to chronic infection begins in the calyces and adjacent parenchyma and progressively extends to involve major segments of the entire kidney. Central necrosis with abscess formation may coalesce to produce large necrotic areas within the kidney as well as within the perinephric space (*Fig. 7.8*). The lesion is difficult to differentiate from tumour and peri-renal or renal abscess formation.

Clinical features

The clinical picture is one of unresolving infection following acute pyelonephritis. The acutely ill patients are often diabetic and ureteric obstruction may be demonstrated. Loin pain, fever, malaise, positive urine culture usually for *E. coli* or *P. mirabilis* and leucocytosis are present.

Investigations and diagnosis

A plain abdominal X-ray may reveal an enlarged kidney with indistinct margins and usually stone disease or calcification. The diagnosis is usually apparent on ultrasound and confirmed by CT scan, particularly with the presence of an associated obstructing stone. Ultrasound reveals a complex mass with cystic and solid components. The diffuse condition involves a majority of the kidney with enlargement and patchy hypoechoic areas, which are difficult to differentiate from tumour. CT provides the best imaging to demonstrate the extent of the renal and peri-renal extension. There is loss of normal architecture with inhomogeneous enhancement along with central necrotic areas of decreased enhancement. Calyceal distortion and obstruction are related to stone disease. Differentiation from tumour is difficult when the process presents as a solid or complex mass infiltrating the kidney and peri-renal space.

Ultrasound or CT-guided needle biopsy of the lesion is frequently not helpful because of the extent of inflammation and necrosis.

Fig. 7.8:
CT scan showing right-sided xanthogranulomatous pyelonephritis.

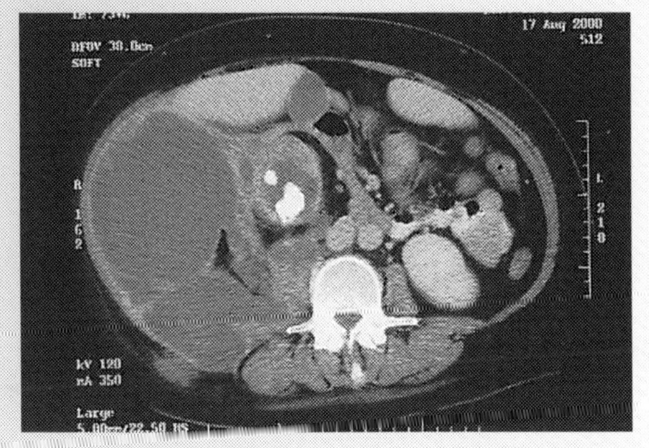

Treatment

Treatment depends on the extent of the necrosis and gas-forming infection within the kidney. Immediate exploration with nephrectomy is usually necessary. Antibiotics to treat infection, control of diabetes and relief of obstructive uropathy are essential. Drainage of the necrotic area with preservation of the kidney is possible if the infection is localized to a segment of the kidney.

Complications

The severity of the infective process may lead to septicaemia which can be life-threatening.

Peri-renal abscess may be present which in turn may lead to fistula formation.

Emphysematous pyelonephritis

Pathology

Emphysematous pyelonephritis occurs as a gas-forming necrotizing pyelonephritis, usually associated with diabetes and resulting from thrombosis of the intra-renal vessels.

Clinical

Emphysematous pyelonephritis is a progression of acute pyelonephritis in the diabetic with impaired resistance to infection and many of the presenting features are similar. Anaerobic metabolism of *E. coli* in the necrotic kidney produces hydrogen and nitrogen gases, which form as patchy collections within the parenchyma (*Fig. 7.9*).

Investigations and treatment

These are similar to those for xanthogranulomatous pyelonephritis. Antibiotics may be effective, but nephrectomy may be necessary.

Fig. 7.9:
CT scan showing emphysematous pyelonephritis with retroperitoneal gas around the right kidney.

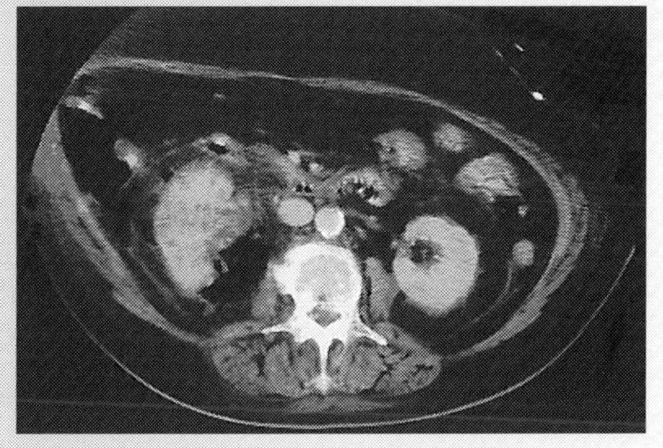

Complications

Renal abscess and perinephric abscess are frequently associated with emphysematous pyelonephritis. In some cases the process may progress to cause necrosis of the entire kidney.

Malacoplakia

Pathology

Malacoplakia is a rare focal chronic inflammatory disorder in patients with chronic illness, immunosuppression or immune deficiency. The diagnosis is made pathologically by demonstrating the presence of characteristic large foamy macrophages and the pathognomonic small basophilic Michaelis–Gutmann bodies.

Clinical

Malacoplakia may involve any system including the urinary tract. Urinary malacoplakia usually involves the bladder, the site where it was first described; however, it occasionally involves the kidney. Urinary tract infection is usually present, typically *E. Coli*.

Investigations

An intravenous pyelogram reveals an enlarged kidney with displacement or distortion of the collecting system. Urinary calculi are rare, a feature distinguishing it from xanthogranulomatous pyelonephritis. Ultrasound reveals a hypoechoic mass, which may have complex cystic change. On CT scan, malacoplakia presents as a localized solid non-enhancing mass lesion.

Treatment

Treatment involves treating any urinary infection and general supportive care.

Key points

- Urinary tract infection is the most common bacterial infection of humans of all ages.
- The symptoms of cystitis are frequency, urgency and pain.
- Examination of the urine is still the key investigation for UTI.
- Bacterial adhesins produced by pili on the bacterial surface are important in pathogenesis.
- The common pathogens are *E. coli*, *Strep. faecalis*, *Proteus* sp., *Pseudomonas* sp. and *Klebsiella* sp.
- Ascending infection causes pyelonephritis: loin pain, fever and malaise.
- Obstruction, stones and infection are intimately linked in cause and effect.
- Chronic bladder irritation from any cause (but especially schistosomiasis) can lead to squamous cell carcinoma of the bladder.
- Genitourinary tuberculosis is common in most parts of the world and is still seen in the West.
- Prostatitis and epididymitis are a major cause of morbidity and time off work in men.

Cases

1. A 20-year-old female student had no significant urinary problems before she was 17 years old. In the last 3 years she has presented on five occasions with dysuria, sometimes with associated haematuria. The MSU specimens have pus cells with a profuse growth of *E. coli* on each occasion.
   (a) How would you investigate her?
   (b) Do you think she needs cystoscopy?
   (c) How would you treat her?
   (d) What difference would it make if the patient was male?

2. A 45-year-old agricultural engineer has just returned from East Africa and has developed symptoms of cystitis and haematuria. He said he had enjoyed swimming in the local lake. Urine cultures are negative.
   (a) Which investigations would you undertake?
   (b) What might cystoscopy show?
   (c) How would you treat him?
   (d) Which complications might ensue?

3. A 73-year-old diabetic woman is admitted with septicaemia and right loin pain and lower urinary tract symptoms.
   (a) How would you manage her in the initial stages?
   (b) What is your differential diagnosis?
   (c) Which further investigations would you do?
   (d) How would you treat her in the longer term?

Answers

1. (a) Apart from the urine examinations she needs an ultrasound scan to exclude upper tract abnormality or urinary retention.
   (b) Cystoscopy is debatable. It should be done for haematuria in the absence of infection, or for any abnormality seen on ultrasound, or if residual urine is present, when a urethral dilatation may be helpful.
   (c) She needs to follow all the hygiene advice as outlined in *Table 7.5*. If the symptoms are related to intercourse an appropriate antibiotic post-intercourse may be helpful. Long-term antibiotics should be reserved for more frequent infections in the absence of any treatable cause.
   (d) Men should be investigated after their **first** UTI with ultrasound, KUB X-ray and flow rates.
2. (a) He needs imaging of his urinary tract in the form of an ultrasound scan and IVU. As the history is suggestive of schistosomiasis (swimming in infected waters) one may find eggs in the urine on microscopy.
   (b) Cystoscopy may show fine yellow sand-like particles under the mucosa.
   (c) Praziquantel in 2 or 3 doses for a single day is effective and has a very low toxicity.
   (d) If the treatment is successful he is unlikely to suffer any complications. Those who live in an endemic area and are untreated will be at risk from long-term irritation and fibrosis of the bladder which in turn may lead to squamous cell cancer of the bladder requiring a cystectomy, or a contracted shrunken bladder with debilitating lower urinary tract symptoms.

3. (a) Her major problem is septicaemia probably associated with diabetes which may be out of control. She needs to be resuscitated and given maximal cardiovascular support. Blood and urine cultures should be taken and intravenous antibiotics given. Her diabetes needs to be brought under control.
   (b) It is likely that the problem is associated with the kidney as she has loin pain and lower urinary tract symptoms. A total of 75% of upper urinary tact infections are associated with lower urinary tract infections, and this associated with loin pain makes it the most likely diagnosis. However, be aware of other possibilities, such as perforated appendicitis, cholecystitis, perforation of the caecum from large bowel obstruction (which could be on the left side, with a competent ileo-caecal valve causing gross distension of the caecum) or even perforated duodenal ulcer with gastric fluid tracting down the right paracolic gutter.
   (c) After the initial investigations a CT urogram will confirm renal pathology.
   (d) This may be acute pyelonephritis with no stone obstruction or other pathology in which case intravenous and then oral antibiotics for several weeks should solve the problem. Pyonephrosis will need draining by nephrostomy or J stent, and a stone needs treating when the infection has settled down. Occasionally the pus is too thick to drain and in this case, or if the kidney is non-functioning, open surgery and a nephrectomy may be necessary.

Further reading

Gillenwater J., Grayhack J.T., Howards S.S. and Duckett, J.W. (1996). *Adult and Paediatric Urology*. 3rd ed. Mosby, St Louis.

Whitfield H.N., Hendry W.F., Kirby R.S. and Duckett J.W. (1998) *Textbook of Genitourinary Surgery*. 2nd ed. Blackwell Science, Oxford.

Resnick M.D. and Novick A.C. (1995) *Urology Secrets*. Hanley & Belfus, Philadelphia.

Luzzi G. (1996) The prostatitis syndromes. *Int J STD & AIDS* 7: 471–478.

CHAPTER 8

Stone disease

Introduction

Urinary stone disease has plagued mankind for centuries. Long before effective treatment was available reference to urinary stones may be found in ancient literature. The oldest stone discovered to date was found in a prehistoric tomb at El Amara amongst the pelvic bones of a teenage boy. It was thought to be a bladder stone dated at over 7000 years old. Historically bladder stones appear to have been endemic in many civilizations and are still prevalent in many regions of the world including the Middle East and northern Africa. In industrialized countries however there was a rise in the incidence of upper tract stones at the turn of the nineteenth century and conversely bladder stones became less common.

There is no doubt that urolithiasis is a significant worldwide problem accounting for a considerable degree of morbidity and mortality in the population. Despite criticism of the studies looking into the prevalence of stone disease it is clear that it is common (1% to 13% of the population in the developed world) with wide geographical variability. Clearly dietary factors play an important role in the site and type of stone formation but detailed epidemiological studies have identified a wide variety of aetiological factors in stone formation (*Table 8.1*).

In recent years the treatment of urinary stones has been completely revolutionized and although lithotomy ('cutting for stone') was historically the only treatment option available it is now unusual for a patient to undergo an open operation as first line treatment. This chapter summarizes the current concepts of aetiology of urinary stones and outlines the clinical features of the condition along with a review of the modern treatment of urinary stone disease.

Table 8.1: Possible aetiological factors involved in the formation of urinary stones

Age
Sex
Hereditary factors and familial disposition
Geography and climate
Drinking habits and diet
Socio-economic factors
Endemic bladder stones

Aetiology and risk factors

Many theories have been proposed to explain the underlying reasons why stones (calculi) develop but none in isolation have been able to answer fully the questions concerning stone formation. It is highly likely that stone disease arises from a combination and interaction of multiple factors. Some of these are well recognized but many are still unknown.

Nucleation theory: A small crystal or foreign body promotes the crystallization and growth of a crystal lattice in urine, which is supersaturated with a crystallizing salt.

Stone matrix theory: A matrix of organic urinary proteins (albumin, mucoproteins etc.) provides a framework for the deposition of crystals.

Inhibition of crystallization theory: There are several urinary substances (magnesium, citrate etc.) which have been demonstrated to inhibit the crystallization of salts in urine. If these are in low concentration or absent in urine then there will be an increased tendency towards stone formation.

Obstruction: stones tend to form at sites of obstruction. Examples would include a renal calyceal diverticulum, a ureterocele, an obstructed bladder or an obstructed prostatic duct.

It is recognized that all three of these processes are likely to be involved in stone formation. After initial crystal nucleation larger crystal aggregates will form providing that some or all of these abnormalities are present in combination with supersaturation of the urine with the salt of the stone-forming crystal. In addition to these factors stones are more likely to form in patients with metabolic abnormalities, making supersaturation of the urine more likely or anatomical abnormalities resulting in urinary stasis with chronic infection.

Several different theories exist as to the actual site of stone formation within the kidney. Deposition of calcium on the basement membrane of collecting tubules or papillae may occur and are referred to as **Randall's plaques**. Alternatively it has been suggested that precipitates of calcium arise within the renal lymphatics, breaking down the membrane separating the lymphatics from the collecting system (**theory of Carr**). Deposition of calcium and cellular debris may occur within the tubules of the collecting system before propagating into larger tubules. This process is known as **intranephronic calculosis**.

Urinary stone disease, as previously mentioned is often related to **metabolic disorders** that result in increased concentration of substances in the urine that constitute stone composition. Not surprisingly many of these conditions relate to calcium metabolism but other rarer conditions may also result in stone disease and certainly any patient who forms stones on a recurrent basis or has a family predisposition to stone formation should be fully investigated for the presence of a metabolic disorder.

Calcium is of course one of the most common constituents of urinary stones and it is therefore not surprising that conditions affecting urinary calcium concentration may be associated with stone formation. Calcium is absorbed from the duodenum and upper jejunum with the aid of a vitamin D-dependent protein. In addition the interaction of vitamin D with parathyroid hormone seems to be essential for calcium absorption.

Absorptive hypercalciuria is the most common abnormality detected in patients with calcium oxalate stones and is present in about 60% of such patients. These patients are thought to have an altered intestinal response to vitamin D leading to increased absorption of calcium, hypercalcaemia and decreased parathyroid secretion. The basis of treatment is to limit calcium and sodium intake in the diet (sodium is known to assist calcium absorption from the gastrointestinal tract), increase dietary fibre that binds to calcium and prevents absorption and increased hydration. Cellulose phosphate may be administered which exchanges sodium for calcium within the gastrointestinal tract and thus reduces calcium absorption and orthophosphates reduce urinary calcium excretion and increase urinary pyrophosphate and citrate excretion. These are both potent inhibitors of calcium stone formation in the urine.

Renal hypercalciuria arises when the kidneys are unable to conserve calcium and is found in about 10% of stone-forming patients. Patients develop hypocalcaemia with increased parathyroid secretion and gastrointestinal calcium absorption. Treatment involves the administration of thiazide diuretics that decrease calcium excretion and also increase urinary zinc and magnesium levels that may enhance the effect.

Hyperparathyroidism is a relatively uncommon condition that accounts for 6% of patients with urinary stone disease. It is more common in females and is recognized by the finding of hypercalcaemia on routine blood analysis. Excessive levels of parathyroid hormone are secreted from the parathyroid glands due to a hormone-secreting adenoma or more rarely carcinoma. This results in increased absorption of calcium from the gastrointestinal tract and resorption from bones. Secondary parathyroidism occurs in response to renal hypercalciuria and tertiary hyperparathyroidism may result when an adenoma arises as a result of chronic overactivity within the parathyroid gland. **Hypercalcaemia** may also be associated with Cushing's disease, myeloma, metastatic cancer, hyperthyroidism etc. and subsequently cause urinary calculi. Patients with **sarcoidosis** usually form mixed calcium stones containing oxalate and phosphate. Hypercalciuria arises in response to increased sensitivity to vitamin D_3 and may be treated with corticosteroids.

Renal tubular acidosis is usually classified into three distinct types one of which is associated with urinary stone formation. Type I renal tubular acidosis occurs as an autosomal dominant condition but can also arise spontaneously. The condition is more common in females and about 70% of patients will form calcium stones. These patients cannot acidify their urine below a pH of 6.0 and have decreased excretion of bicarbonate, potassium and citrate in their urine. They also develop hypercalciuria, metabolic acidosis and subsequent bone demineralization. The stones are usually pure calcium phosphate and patients are prone to nephrocalcinosis (stone formation within the cortical tubular structure of the kidney). Patients are advised to drink plenty of fluid and may require sodium bicarbonate or sodium potassium citrate to alkalinize the urine. Type II and type IV are not associated with urinary stones.

Hyperoxaluria is an important consideration in the urinary stone formation given that 70% to 80% of urinary calculi identified comprise of calcium oxalate. **Primary hyperoxaluria** is a general term describing two rare genetic disorders characterized by excessive production of oxalic acid that results in recurrent calcium oxalate neprolithiasis and nephrocalcinosis. Patients often present with the clinical features of urinary calculi and progress to death in their early twenties. Oxalic acid is an end product of metabolism and disorders of its breakdown result in hyperoxaluria. Type I hyperoxaluria is caused by a deficiency of alanine:glycoxalate aminotransferase. Treatment is aimed at lowering oxalate excretion by dietary control, decelerating oxalate synthesis with pyridoxine administration, increasing fluid intake and increasing inhibition of calcium oxalate crystallization with magnesium oxide/hydroxide. Type II hyperoxaluria is extremely rare and once again inherited as an autosomal recessive condition. It is caused by a deficiency of D-glycerate dehydrogenase (DGD). It tends to be less severe than type I hyperoxaluria and first manifests in later childhood.

Uric acid stones account for about 10% of urinary calculi and interestingly humans and Dalmatian dogs are the only mammals known to suffer with the condition. Uric acid is an end product of purine metabolism and is very insoluble in acidic water. As urine becomes more acidic more uric acid will become insoluble and thus lead to stone formation. Uric acid stones arise in patients with an **idiopathic** form of the disease with normal levels of serum and urinary uric acid. In other patients **hyperuricaemia** is associated with a metabolic abnormality such as primary gout or the Lesch-Nyhan syndrome. About 25% of patients with gout develop uric acid urinary stones. Hyperuricaemia also occurs in patients with myeloproliferative disorders and urinary uric acid secretion is raised in patients receiving chemotherapy. Chronic diarrhoea may be associated with the formation of uric acid stones especially in patients with ileostomies and rarely hyperuricosuria may occur in patients who are normouricaemic. This condition may be seen as a side effect of thiazide diuretics and salicylate therapy. Treatment is based upon adequate hydration, dietary control and alkalinization of the urine with sodium bicarbonate. Allopurinol, the xanthine oxidase inhibitor can be used in patients to prevent stone formation but may be associated with skin rash, fever etc. Pure uric acid stones are radiolucent and care is therefore needed in the choice of investigation in patients with this condition.

Cystinuria occurs due to an inherited defect in the transport of the amino acids cystine, lysine, arginine and ornithine. Cystine is insoluble and therefore excessive concentrations within urine lead to cystine lithiasis. It is inherited as an autosomal recessive condition and diagnosis is based upon the finding of cystine crystals within the urine that are present in up to 80% of patients. Some patients exhibit mild or heterozygous cystinuria and rarely excrete enough cystine in their urine to form pure cystine stones. However calcium oxalate stones are common in this group of patients and it is thought that cystine aggregates may form a nidus on which calcium oxalate can then precipitate. Patients usually present after puberty but the stones are often not clearly visible on plain radiographs having a ground glass appearance thus leading to delays in diagnosis. Treatment consists of hydration, alkalinization of the urine and the use of cystine-binding drugs such as penicillamine.

Hypocitraturia is said to be a co-existent factor in the formation of urinary calculi in up to 60% of patients. Citrate is known to inhibit crystallization of calcium oxalate and calcium phosphate and may also prevent crystal nucleation. Potassium citrate may reduce the risk of new stone formation.

Urinary stone formation is also common in the presence of **chronic urinary tract infection**. These stones are twice as common in women as in men and account for 15% of all urinary calculi. They are often large and fill the pelvicalyceal system, giving the characteristic '**staghorn**' appearances. Chemically, they comprise of a mixture of magnesium ammonium phosphate and calcium apatite, referred to as triple phosphate or struvite stones. The stones usually arise in the presence of 'urea-splitting' organisms within the urine, typically *Proteus* species. These organisms alkalinize the urine above pH 7.0, causing precipitation of urinary calcium and other ions. Treatment involves eradicating the urinary tract infection and stone removal and occasionally urease inhibitors such as acetohydroxamic acid have been employed with some success.

Clinical features

Most urinary stones are likely to form in the kidney and then pass through the ureters, bladder and urethra depending on their size and other anatomical factors. The symptoms caused by these stones will thus depend upon their size, position and the presence of complicating factors such as infection.

Most patients will present with isolated symptoms of **loin pain**, with or without **haematuria**. Symptoms related to **urinary tract infection** such as dysuria, urinary frequency and fever may also occur. Stones should be suspected if a patient is suffering recurrent UTIs. Many renal stones are **asymptomatic** and identified when investigations are performed as a result of other clinical conditions. Stones situated in renal calyces may be small and asymptomatic but occasionally present after a single episode of relatively painless haematuria. When they become big enough to obstruct the flow of urine from a calyx they may cause flank pain, haematuria and recurrent infection. Stones that become lodged at the pelviureteric junction may cause severe loin pain associated with **nausea and vomiting**. If there is associated infection patients will quickly become unwell with evidence of pyelonephritis or septicaemia in more severe cases.

When smaller stones pass down from the kidney to the ureter patients may complain of typical '**ureteric colic**' (see also Chapter 3). The pain originates in the loin, comes in waves of severity often lasting several minutes and radiates into the scrotum and testis in the male and labia in the female. Stones typically become lodged at three main sites in the ureter, the pelviureteric junction, the point at which the ureter crosses the iliac vessels and finally as the ureter enters the bladder at the vesicoureteric junction. More severe and consistent pain with or without haematuria may occur if the stone becomes 'stuck' at any of these sites. Once again superimposed urinary tract infection can complicate ureteric colic and lead to sepsis in severe cases.

As the stone nears the bladder **filling lower urinary tract symptoms** will become more severe due to irritation of the trigone of the bladder although once the stone is passed into the bladder the symptoms may settle (*Fig. 8.1*). Patients may or may not notice passing a stone through the urethra. Larger

Fig. 8.1:
A small stone is seen near to the ureterovesical junction in a patient presenting with classical 'ureteric colic'.

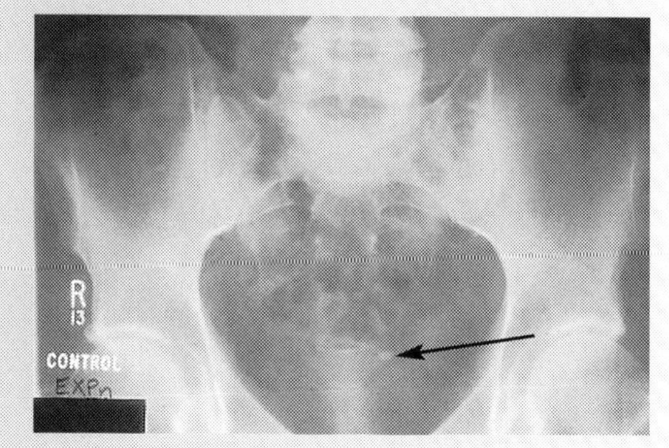

stones may of course be more painful to void and be associated with haematuria due to trauma to the urethral urothelium.

Bladder stones will present with increasing filling lower urinary tract symptoms and recurrent urinary tract infection. Voiding may be interrupted in a variable manner as the stone falls into the bladder outlet causing intermittent obstruction and severe '**stranguary**' may be associated with the presence of a large bladder stone (*Fig. 8.2*). Rarely, a patient who has passed a sizeable stone into the urethra may present in **painful retention** of urine.

Non-specific symptoms may be associated with the presence of urinary stones in patients with chronic urolithiasis. **Failure to thrive** in a child may indicate the presence of **chronic urinary tract infection** with stones and the highly variable patterns of abdominal pain mean that the diagnosis should be considered in all patients with acute abdominal pain even if gastrointestinal pathology seems more likely on initial assessment. The presence of an abdominal aortic aneurysm may initiate symptoms similar to those of renal or ureteric colic and should be carefully considered in patients presenting in this way.

Fig. 8.2:
A large bladder stone identified on a plain radiograph of the abdomen and pelvis.

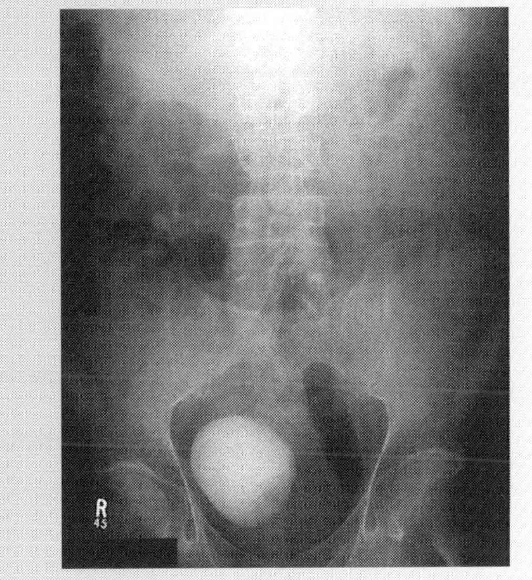

Physical examination often reveals a pale patient in severe distress with considerable pain. The patient may well be **vomiting** with **tachypnoea** and a **tachycardia**. The presence of **pyrexia** should be established at an early stage as a sign of **sepsis**. In comparison to a patient with peritonitis who will invariably remain still, the patient with renal or ureteric colic is often **restless**, moving around excessively in an effort to find a more comfortable position and this clinical observation is a useful diagnostic sign in cases where symptoms are not clear cut. The abdomen should be carefully palpated for signs of localized tenderness and to rule out other causes of acute abdominal pain. As mentioned before the presence of a pulsatile mass should raise the suspicion of an abdominal aortic aneurysm

When assessing a patient clinically with a suspected diagnosis of urinary tract stones always bear in mind that a potentially more serious gastrointestinal, gynaecological or vascular diagnosis may be present and these possibilities must be excluded especially where conservative treatment is likely to be initiated for presumed stone disease.

Investigations

The investigations commonly employed in the identification of urinary tract calculi have been discussed elsewhere. In general terms the goals of investigation are as follows:

(a) To confirm the diagnosis.
(b) Is there evidence of urinary tract infection?
(c) Where is the stone?
(d) How big is the stone?
(e) Is the kidney partially/fully obstructed?
(f) Are there multiple stones present?
(g) What is the relative function of each kidney?
(h) To identify aetiological factors associated with the formation of urinary stones e.g. metabolic disorders, anatomical abnormalities.

Urinalysis is mandatory for all patients suspected of having urinary stones. In the acute presentation the presence of **microscopic or macroscopic haematuria** will suggest urinary tract pathology. Perhaps of more importance is the situation encountered where a patient presents with clinical features of ureteric colic but blood is not identified in the urine. In this situation the diagnosis of urinary stones is unlikely and an alternative explanation for the symptoms should be looked for. Similarly the presence of blood in the urine is not always diagnostic of urinary stone disease. The presence of **pyuria** and **infection** in the urine may suggest an increased risk of sepsis and can alter the approach to management. In the non-acute situation the **pH** of the urine may give clues as to the aetiology of urinary stone disease and the presence of crystals, i.e. uric acid crystals may point to an underlying diagnosis.

Radiological imaging is usually undertaken initially with a **plain X-ray of the kidneys, ureters and bladder (KUB)** and an **ultrasound scan (USS)** of the urinary tract. These investigations will demonstrate the size and position of most urinary tract calculi and demonstrate the presence of upper tract dilatation. **Most (90%) urinary stones are radiopaque and are easily identified on a KUB X-ray** but radiolucent stones such as uric acid stones will usually be seen with USS. **Intravenous urography (IVU)** is now rarely used as a first line investigation in urinary stone disease, excluding the emergency investigation of ureteric colic. IVU may be performed if the diagnosis is not clear from KUB X-ray and USS. In recent years **computerized tomography urography (CTU)** has superseded IVU in the investigation of urinary stones in some centres. It is not only employed in the acute phase but can also be useful in the planning of access etc. to the kidney for percutaneous surgery. CTU is also useful in the investigation of radiolucent stones. Static **renography** can be utilized where knowledge of the relative function of an individual kidney is important. In a patient with a unilateral stag-horn renal calculus, attempted removal of the stone is not indicated where there is little or no function left in the kidney. In this scenario a simple nephrectomy would be a better option.

Metabolic stone screening is undertaken to investigate any possible disorder that predisposes the patient to recurrent stone formation. In addition to routine blood tests for **calcium**, **oxalate and urate**, a **24-hour urine collection** is undertaken to look at abnormal concentrations of stone-forming substances and inhibitors within the urine. Abnormal **amino acid** concentration within the urine may suggest a diagnosis of cystinuria. It is always essential to send any **stones or stone fragments** for analysis as this will also give important aetiological information regarding the nature of stone formation within an individual patient.

Treatment

In the **acute presentation** of urinary stone disease the clinician needs to assess a number of key questions before making a treatment decision:

(a) Is the stone likely to pass spontaneously?
(b) Is there evidence of continuing upper tract obstruction?
(c) Is there evidence of urinary sepsis?
(d) Are there complicating factors present? i.e. solitary kidney, pregnancy etc.

Most stones that are 5 mm or less in diameter have a very good chance of spontaneous passage without the need to intervene: 50% will pass if situated in the upper ureter at presentation and 90% will pass if situated in the distal ureter. Larger stones are less likely to pass spontaneously. Stones are likely to be held up at the pelviureteric junction, the pelvic brim or the vesicoureteric junction but if small will eventually pass through. During this time the patient should be given adequate **analgesia** (for example, diclofenac 50 mg 8-hourly) and carefully counselled to expect more pain as the stone moves. It is not uncommon for patients to suffer continuing pain for several hours after the stone has passed, probably due to oedema within the ureter. Some small stones may not pass spontaneously, either due to irregular morphology or excessive ureteric oedema. Adequate time should be left to allow the stone to pass before resorting to invasive measures to remove the stone, provided that the patient's pain can be controlled with simple analgesics.

If there is clinical evidence of progressive **upper tract obstruction** (non-resolving or increasing pain), of infection (pain and swinging fever) then active intervention is necessary as an emergency even if the stone appears to be small (also see Chapter 3). Under normal circumstances a **nephrostomy** tube can be placed radiologically to decompress the kidney, allowing obstruction to be relieved and infection to settle with intravenous antibiotics etc. Where the patient has a single kidney retrograde **double J ureteric stent** placement should be considered rather than nephrostomy due to risk of damage to the kidney with needle nephrostomy placement.

Renal calculi that fail to pass spontaneously or larger stones will require active intervention. Modern stone treatment involves extracorporeal shock wave lithotripsy (ESWL), endoscopic stone removal or open stone surgery.

ESWL permits fragmentation of renal (and occasionally ureteric and bladder calculi) without the need for direct surgical intervention. ESWL was first used to treat urinary tract calculi in the early 1980s and has since revolutionized stone treatment. In simple terms an acoustic shock wave is generated by the lithotripter apparatus using either electrohydraulic, electromagnetic or piezoelectric energy. The shock wave is then focused on the stone using either ultrasound or image intensification. The strength and frequency of the shock wave can then be altered according to patient tolerability but with most modern lithotripters patients can tolerate treatment on an out-patient basis with minimal analgesia. Post treatment patients are warned that haematuria and pain may occur as stone fragments are passed down the ureter and antibiotics are usually administered to avoid infective complications. Occasionally a 'cloud' of minute stone fragments pass down the ureter collectively causing upper tract obstruction. This phenomenon is referred to as a '**stonestrasse**' and may require the temporary insertion of a double J stent to relieve obstruction and subsequent ureteroscopy to remove the fragments in some cases (*Fig. 8.3*). Limitations to using ESWL to treat renal stones include very large stag-horn calculi (which often require a combination of ESWL and percutaneous renal surgery), patients on anti-coagulant therapy, body habitus (patients with deformed spines etc.), abnormal drainage from the kidney (pelviureteric junction obstruction, horseshoe kidney) or ureter (ureterocele, stricture) and pregnancy.

Percutaneous nephrolithotomy (PCNL) involves the insertion of a nephroscope through a nephrostomy tract to remove a stone from a calyx or the pelvis of the kidney. An ultrasound or pneumatic **intracorporeal lithotripter** can then be used to fragment the stone under direct vision. The advantages of this technique include the lack of a surgical wound to remove the stone with a much quicker recovery period post-operatively. Complications of this procedure include haemorrhage from the nephrostomy tract and prolonged nephrostomy drainage especially if there is distal obstruction present. Large stag-horn calculi may be treated in combination with ESWL but multiple treatments may be necessary to render the patient stone-free.

Fig. 8.3:
A stonestrasse complicating treatment of a renal calculus with ESWL.

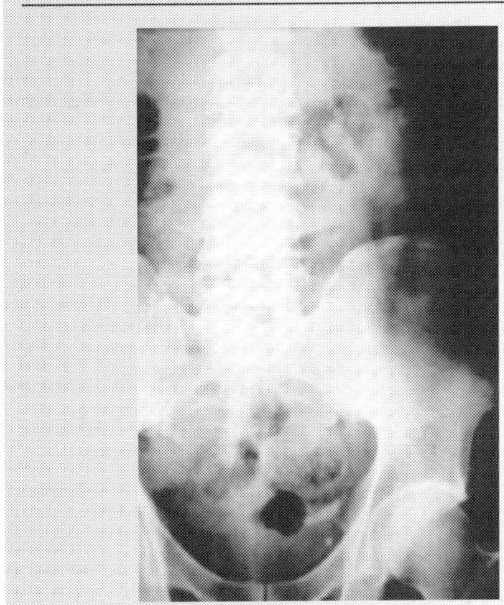

Open nephrolithotomy was once the only available method for removing renal calculi necessitating the use of hypothermic renal surgery and on-table radiographic location of stones. Nowadays <1% of renal stones are removed by open operation and are usually reserved for patients in whom other treatment modalities have been unsuccessful or access to the kidney radiologically or percutaneously is difficult due to body habitus etc. **Partial nephrectomy** may occasionally be necessary if stone clearance proves to be technically impossible and **simple nephrectomy** may be indicated in a poorly or non-functioning kidney, either open or laparoscopic.

Ureteric calculi that have not passed spontaneously can be treated with in-situ ESWL. However many are removed with **ureteroscopy**. Modern rigid and flexible instruments allow excellent access to all sections of the ureter. Intracorporeal lithotripsy, usually pneumatic or laser energy, can be transmitted down the instrument channel of the endoscope to fragment the stone. Stone fragments are then removed using endoscopic forceps or a basket, under direct vision. **Open ureterolithotomy** is now rarely employed in the treatment of ureteric stones although occasionally utilized where ureteric strictures have arisen making access with a ureteroscope difficult.

Dissolution therapy should be considered either in isolation or as an adjunct to stone surgery. The specific treatments employed have been discussed previously with relation to each specific stone type.

Bladder calculi are often treated endoscopically and are crushed using a stone punch or pneumatic lithotripter. For larger bladder calculi **open lithotomy** is often still the treatment of choice.

Prostatic calculi are usually asymptomatic and are only identified when the prostate is imaged either with a plain radiograph or at trans-rectal ultrasonography. They may be seen during endoscopic examination of the prostatic urethra or during a trans-urethral resection of prostate. They are often associated with prostatitis. They usually are formed of calcium phosphate. Occasionally prostatic calculi are extrinsic i.e. primarily formed in other parts of the urinary tract and may cause obstruction to urinary flow within the prostatic urethra during voiding.

Urethral stones are rarely primary and usually become impacted on passage from the bladder. These stones can be removed endoscopically or at open operation where they have formed in a urethral diverticulum.

Key points

- 90% of renal/ureteric calculi are radiopaque.
- Aetiology is multi-factorial and poorly understood.
- In the acute presentation is there evidence of upper tract obstruction in the presence of infection? If so decompress the upper tract urgently.
- 90% of stones ≤ 5 mm in the distal ureter will pass spontaneously.
- Beware the leaking abdominal aortic aneurysm mimicking the presentation of a ureteric stone.
- Remember to investigate metabolic abnormalities especially in recurrent stone formers and children.
- Despite modern treatment options open surgery is still occasionally necessary.

Cases

1. A 24-year-old man presents with right-sided loin pain radiating into his left testicle. He has microscopic haematuria.
   (a) Which investigations would you do?
   (b) How would you treat this man?
   (c) Which complications may arise?
   (d) How would you follow him up?

2. A 64-year-old woman presents with recurrent urinary tract infections and imaging reveals a large stag-horn calculus in her right kidney.
   (a) What is the likely infecting organism?
   (b) What is the likely chemical constituent of the stone?
   (c) Which other investigations would you do and why?
   (d) How would you treat this stone?

3. An 18-year-old man presents with loin pain. A KUB reveals a slightly radiopaque stone overlying the left kidney with a ground-glass appearance.
   (a) What is the likely chemical constituent of this stone?
   (b) Which tests would you do to investigate this further?
   (c) Which treatment would you advise?
   (d) Which other measures might you consider?

Answers

1. (a) KUB and ultrasound of urinary tract. Proceed to CTU if information not adequate on original investigations.
   (b) If he has a small ureteric stone <5 mm then this is likely to pass spontaneously and can be treated spontaneously. He should be given analgesia and encouraged to drink adequate fluids whilst the stone passes. He should be warned that he might suffer from further bouts of severe pain whilst the stone is passing and that this may persist for several days. If the stone is larger then it may require treatment with in-situ ESWL or ureteroscopic stone fragmentation and extraction.
   (c) Upper tract obstruction and/or urinary tract sepsis. This may reqire urgent upper tract decompression with a nephrostomy tube placement or retrograde double J stent insertion.
   (d) When the stone has passed/been removed a follow-up KUB/USS should be performed to look for further stone formation. A metabolic stone screen is undertaken and the patient given advice regarding fluid intake and diet etc.

2. (a) *Proteus mirabilis*. This is a urea-splitting organism which predisposes to large stag-horn calculi by alkalizing the urine.
   (b) Magnesium calcium ammonium phosphate of 'Struvite' stone.
   (c) A DMSA renogram. The reason for performing this investigation is to ascertain the relative function of each kidney prior to treatment.
   (d) If there is good relative function in the right kidney or relatively poor function in the contralateral kidney then treatment should involve antibiotics and a combination of ESWL and PCNL. If there is little or no function in the right kidney then open or laparoscopic nephrectomy would be indicated.

3. (a) Cystine.
   (b) To investigate the stone itself a CTU would be indicated prior to treatment to show the exact position of the stone within the kidney. To further investigate cystinuria a 24 h urine collection is analysed for total cystine content and any stone fragments obtained during treatment sent off for analysis.
   (c) Cystine stones are often very hard and may be resistant to ESWL. PCNL may therefore be necessary. After stone removal the patient should be given advice regarding fluid intake and consideration be given to alkalinization of the urine with sodium bicarbonate. If stone recurrence becomes frequent then administration of penicillamine may be necessary.
   (d) Family screening for cystinuria.

Further reading

Whitfield H.N., Hendry W.F., Kirby R.S. and Duckett J.W. (1998). *Textbook of Genitourinary Surgery*. Second ed. Blackwell Science, Oxford.

Gillenwater J., Grayhack J.T., Howards S.S. and Duckett J.W. (1996). *Adult and Paediatric Urology*. Third ed. Mosby, St. Louis.

Walsh P.C., Retik A.B., Stamey T.A. and Vaughan E.D. (1999). *Campbell's Urology*. Seventh ed. Saunders, Philadelphia.

CHAPTER 9

Urological oncology

Renal tumours

Introduction

Like all neoplasia, renal neoplasia is a genetic disease. It may be hereditary or sporadic, depending on whether the genetic abnormalities are constitutional (germ-line) or somatic (acquired). Tumours may be benign or malignant, primary or secondary. Hereditary tumours tend to appear at a younger age than their sporadic counterparts, and are often multifocal, due to an underlying constitutional genetic abnormality. Malignant epithelial tumours are termed carcinomas; connective tissue tumours are named according to their components, adding their benign (-oma) or malignant (-sarcoma) characterization. For example, a benign tumour composed of blood vessels, fat and smooth muscle is an **angiomyolipoma**; a malignant tumour composed of smooth muscle is a leiomyosarcoma. Sarcomas are rare in the kidney, constituting 1% of all renal neoplasms. Primary renal tumours commonly arise from renal tubular epithelium (**renal cell carcinoma**) or the transitional epithelium of the calyces and renal pelvis (**transitional cell carcinoma**). Less commonly, other epithelium (for example, the glomerulus or juxtaglomerular cells) or connective tissue give rise to tumours. There are two notable additions: the first is the **Wilms' tumour**, which arises from the embryonic mesenchyme of the metanephric blastema; the second is the benign renal **oncocytoma**, thought to arise from cells of the collecting ducts. Secondary renal tumours (metastases) are uncommon; they may spread from the lung. The tumours highlighted are discussed in detail below.

Wilms' tumour (nephroblastoma)

This is a rare childhood tumour, affecting 1 in 10 000 children. However, it represents 80% of all genitourinary tumours affecting children under 15 years. Males and females are equally affected, 20% are familial and 5% are bilateral. A total of 75% present under the age of 5 years.

Pathology and staging

Wilms' tumour is a soft pale grey tumour (it looks like brain). It contains blastemal, epithelial and connective tissue components. Mutation or deletion of both copies of the WT-1 tumour suppressor gene, on chromosome 11p, result in development of this tumour. Affected family members harbour a germ-line mutation, so only one further mutation is required: this helps to explain why hereditary Wilms' tumours tend to develop multifocally and at a slightly younger age than sporadic ones. Tumour staging relates to the relationship of the tumour to the renal capsule, excision margins and local lymph nodes at nephrectomy, as well as the presence of soft tissue (e.g. lung) or bone metastases.

Presentation

A total of 90% have a mass, 33% complain of abdominal or loin pain, 30–50% develop haematuria, 50% are hypertensive and 15% exhibit other anomalies, such as hemihypertrophy, aniridia and cryptorchidism (undescended testes).

Investigations

The first-line investigation for a child with an abdominal mass or haematuria is ultrasound, which will reveal a renal tumour. An IVU may show pelvicalyceal distortion due to compression by the tumour, but may be unhelpful if the kidney is non-functioning. Further information to help with diagnosis and staging is obtained by CT scanning. An X-ray or CT of the chest is necessary for staging Wilms' tumour.

Treatment and prognosis

Children with renal tumours should be managed by a specialist paediatric oncology centre. A staging nephrectomy, with or without pre-operative or post-operative chemotherapy, remains the mainstay of treatment. The chemotherapy most frequently used is actinomycin D, vincristine and doxorubicin. Survival is generally good, at 92% overall, ranging from 55% to 97% according to stage and histology.

Renal cell carcinoma (RCC)

Renal cell carcinoma, also known as hypernephroma since it was erroneously believed to originate in the adrenal gland, is the commonest of renal tumours, accounting for 3% of all adult malignancies and 85% of renal malignancies. In 1997, 3033 patients died because of metastatic RCC in the UK. It is also known as clear cell carcinoma (as it commonly appears microscopically) and Grawitz tumour.

Risk factors

Males are affected twice as commonly as females. Studies have shown an association with cigarette smoking, asbestos exposure, the analgesic phenacitin and exposure to thorium dioxide. Anatomical risk factors include polycystic kidneys and horseshoe kidneys. The majority of patients present in their sixth and seventh decades, although patients younger than 50 years present, particularly those with the rare hereditary form – von Hippel Lindau (VHL) syndrome. 50% of individuals with this autosomal dominant syndrome, characterized by phaeochromocytoma, renal and pancreatic cysts and cerebellar haemangioblastoma, develop RCC (*Fig. 9.1*).

Fig. 9.1: A renal CT scan showing multiple left renal cysts and two right renal tumours. This patient has the von Hippel Lindau syndrome.

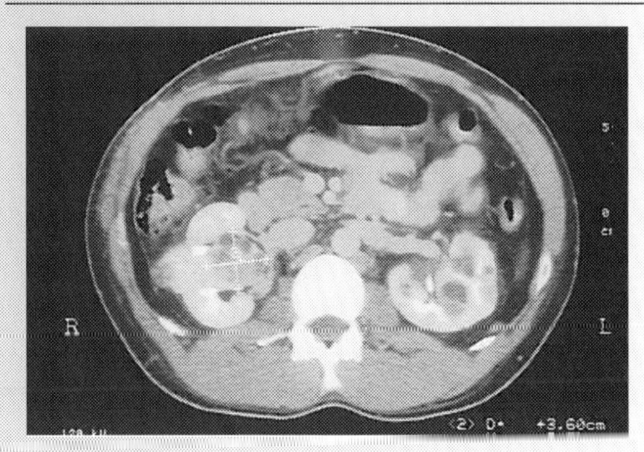

Pathology and staging

RCC is an adenocarcinoma, arising from renal tubular cells. Usually solid with a tan colour, they may contain cysts and occasionally be predominantly cystic. Up to 5% are multifocal. RCC has a particular tendency to grow into the renal vein and occasionally to the inferior vena cava (IVC) and right atrium. The VHL tumour suppressor gene, on chromosome 3p, is inactivated in VHL patients and is mutated in the majority of sporadic RCCs. Staging is by the TNM system.

Presentation

50% of patients present with haematuria; 40% develop loin pain; in 40% of patients, the renal tumour is an incidental finding on abdominal ultrasonography; 30% of patients notice a mass; 25% have symptoms or signs of metastatic disease (e.g. haemoptysis, weight loss); only 10% of patients exhibit the classic triad of haematuria, pain and mass. Less common presenting features include acute varicocele, due to obstruction of the testicular vein by tumour within the left renal vein (5%), and paraneoplastic syndromes (*Table 9.1*), due to ectopic hormone secretion by the tumour (5%).

Investigations

The first-line investigation for a patient with haematuria, loin pain or a mass includes abdominal ultrasound, which will reveal a renal mass or complex cyst. If a renal cyst has a solid intracystic element, an irregular or calcified wall, it is regarded as potentially malignant and consideration should be given to radical excision. Further information and staging is by CT scanning the chest and abdomen with IV contrast administration. This will also provide evidence that the contralateral kidney

Table 9.1:
Paraneoplastic syndromes

Syndrome associated with RCC	Cause
Anaemia	Haematuria, chronic disease
Polycythaemia	Ectopic secretion of erythropoietin
Hypertension	Ectopic secretion of renin
Hypoglycaemia	Ectopic secretion of insulin
Cushing's	Ectopic secretion of ACTH
Hypercalcaemia	Ectopic secretion of parathyroid hormone-like substance
Gynaecomastia, amenorrhoea, reduced libido, baldness	Ectopic secretion of gonadotrophins
Hepatic dysfunction (Stauffer's syndrome)	Unknown
Pyrexia/night sweats	Unknown

Fig. 9.2:
A renal CT scan showing a right upper pole tumour and tumour within the expanded inferior vena cava.

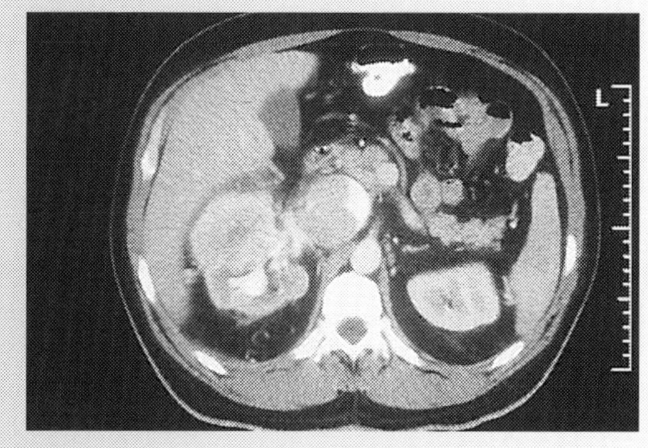

is functioning (*Fig. 9.2*). If required, the IVC is best imaged with MRI.

Urine cytology and culture should be normal. Full blood count may reveal polycythaemia or anaemia. Serum creatinine and electrolytes are recommended, together with calcium and liver function tests.

Needle biopsy is not recommended, since the result may be misleading.

Treatment and prognosis

If the renal mass appears to be confined to the kidney or perinephric fascia and non-metastatic, **radical nephrectomy** is the recommended treatment, with curative intent. This involves excision of the kidney, adrenal gland and peri-renal tissue usually by a transperitoneal approach. If the tumour is small (under 4 cm), or bilateral, or if the patient has a single functioning kidney, **partial nephrectomy** is the best option. Complications of the latter include failure of complete excision of the tumour(s) and urinary leak from the collecting system. Patients with VHL, who often develop multifocal and bilateral RCC, may eventually require renal replacement therapy. **Follow-up** should include periodic radiological assessments of the chest, and if the RCC was locally advanced, surveillance of the renal bed using ultrasound or CT is recommended.

Patients with **metastatic disease** have a generally poor prognosis. The primary tumour should be removed if it is causing symptoms and the patient is fit. Renal artery embolization is another option if haematuria is a problem. Occasionally, the metastasis is solitary and potentially resectable, together with the primary tumour. RCC is rarely radiosensitive or responsive to chemotherapy. Multiple metastases show a 30% response rate after systemic immunotherapy, survival is possibly improved by nephrectomy. Agents include interleukin-2 and interferon-alpha, although toxicity can be severe.

5-year survival:

Organ-confined	T1,2	80%
Locally advanced	T3a	60–70%
Locally advanced/IVC	T3b,c, T4	50%
Lymph node involvement	N+	20%
Pulmonary or bone metastasis	M+	10%

Transitional cell carcinoma (TCC) of the renal pelvis

This is uncommon, accounting for 8% of renal malignancies and 5% of all transitional cell carcinomas. Risk factors are similar to those of TCC in the bladder (see page 96). Males are affected three times as commonly as females, incidence increases with age, smoking confers a two-fold risk and there are various occupational causes. TCC does not have a genetic hereditary form.

Pathology and staging

The tumour usually has a papillary structure and arises within the renal pelvis, less frequently in one of the calyces or ureter. Histologically, features of TCC are present, described below. Staging is by the TNM classification. It is bilateral in 2–4%.

Presentation

90% of patients present with painless total haematuria; 30% have loin pain, often caused by clots passing down the ureter ('clot colic'). A synchronous bladder TCC will be present in 10%; at follow-up, half of these patients will develop a metachronous bladder TCC and 2% will develop contralateral upper tract TCC.

Investigations

Diagnosis is usually made on urine cytology and IVU, respectively revealing malignant cells and a filling defect in the renal pelvis (*Fig. 9.3*) or ureter. If doubt exists, retrograde ureterography is indicated. Ultrasound is excellent for detecting the more common renal parenchymal tumours, but not sensitive at detecting tumours of the renal pelvis. Hence, if the ultrasound and cystoscopy are normal during the investigation of haematuria, an IVU is recommended. TNM staging is obtained by contrast-enhanced abdominal CT, chest X-ray and occasionally a bone scan.

Fig. 9.3:
An IVU showing a filling defect in the right renal pelvis which was a transitional cell carcinoma. Incidentally, there is a partial duplication of the left ureter.

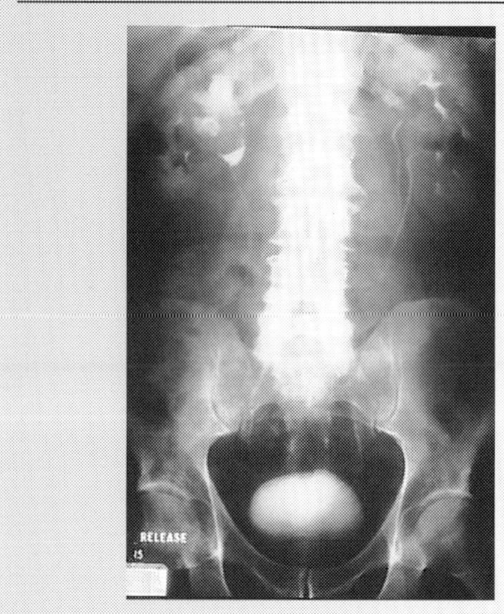

Treatment and prognosis

If staging indicates non-metastatic disease, the gold standard treatment with curative intent is **nephroureterectomy**, approached using a long transperitoneal midline incision or two separate incisions. The ipsilateral ureter is taken because of the 50% incidence of subsequent ureteric stump recurrence. An alternative option for patients with a single functioning kidney, bilateral disease or those who are unfit, is ureterorenoscopic resection or ablation of the tumour. This is less likely to be curative, however. **Follow-up** should include cystoscopies and IVUs. In metastatic disease, combination chemotherapy using cyclophosphamide, methotrexate and vincristine is associated with a 30% total or partial response at the expense of moderate toxicity. Palliative surgery or renal artery embolization may be necessary for troublesome haematuria. Radiotherapy is generally ineffective.

5-year survival:

Organ-confined	T1,2	60–100%
Locally advanced	T3,4	20–50%
Node-positive	N+	15%
Pulmonary, bone metastases	M+	10%

Oncocytoma

This is uncommon, accounting for 3–5% of renal tumours. Males are twice as commonly affected as females. They can occur simultaneously with renal cell carcinoma in up to 33% of cases.

Pathology

Oncocytomas are spherical, capsulated and brown or tan-colour. Half contain a central scar. Histologically, they comprise aggregates of eosinophilic cells, packed with mitochondria. Mitoses are rare and they are considered benign, not known to metastasize. There is often loss of the Y chromosome.

Presentation

Oncocytomas often present as an incidental finding, or with loin pain or haematuria.

Investigations

Oncocytomas usually cannot be distinguished radiologically from RCC; they may co-exist with RCC. Rarely, they exhibit a spoke-wheel pattern on CT scanning, caused by a central scar (*Fig. 9.4*). Percutaneous biopsy is not recommended since it often leads to continuing uncertainty about the diagnosis.

Fig. 9.4:
A renal CT scan showing a well-defined left renal tumour that was an oncocytoma. Careful inspection reveals the impression of the central scar characteristic of these tumours.

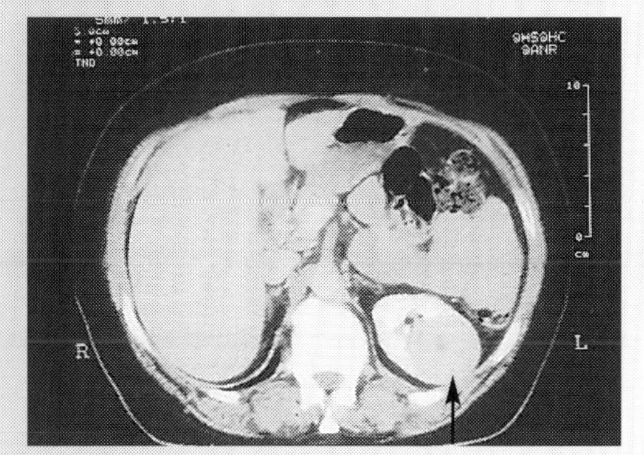

Treatment

Radical or partial nephrectomy is indicated.

Angiomyolipoma (AML)

These hamartomas occur sporadically, mostly in females, or in association with tuberous sclerosis (TS). This is a hereditary autosomal dominant syndrome, characterized by mental retardation, epilepsy, adenoma sebaceum, and other benign hamartomas. In TS, tumours are frequently multifocal and bilateral.

Pathology

AML, as its name suggests, is composed of blood vessels, muscle and fat. Macroscopically, it looks like a well-circumscribed lump of fat. If solitary, they are more frequently found in the right kidney. They are always considered benign.

Presentation

AMLs frequently present as incidental findings on ultrasound or CT scans. They may present with painless total haematuria, which may occasionally be severe and potentially life-threatening.

Investigations

Ultrasound reflects from fat, hence a characteristic bright echo-pattern. This does not cast an 'acoustic shadow' beyond, helping to distinguish an AML from a calculus. CT shows this fatty tumour as a low-density mass, often septated (*Fig. 9.5*). Measurement of the diameter is relevant to treatment.

Treatment

Asymptomatic AMLs can be observed if they measure less than 4 cm, since they rarely bleed. If they are greater than 4 cm, or bleeding, nephrectomy is indicated. Occasionally, emergency nephrectomy is life-saving. In patients with TS, in whom multiple bilateral lesions are present, conservative surgery should be attempted.

Bladder tumours

Bladder cancer is the second most common urological malignancy, accounting for 5108 deaths in the UK in 1997. However, there are 13 000 new cases

Fig. 9.5:
A renal CT scan showing large bilateral fatty tumours consistent with angiomyolipomas. There is little evidence of normal kidney tissue in this film.

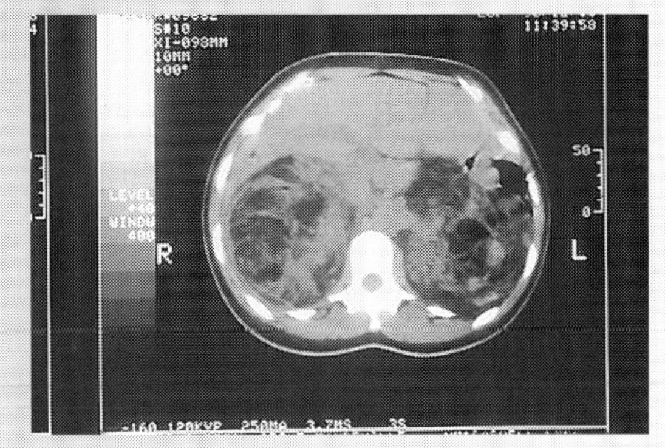

per year, indicating that the majority of patients die with, rather than of, bladder cancer.

Risk factors

Men are three times more likely to develop the disease, increasing with age. No evidence for a hereditary genetic aetiology exists, although black people have a lower incidence than white people.

Environmental carcinogens, found in urine, are the major cause of bladder cancer. Factors causing chronic inflammation of bladder mucosa are also implicated.

Smoking is the major cause of bladder cancer in the developed world. Cigarette smoke contains the carcinogens 4-aminobiphenyl and 2-naphthylamine.

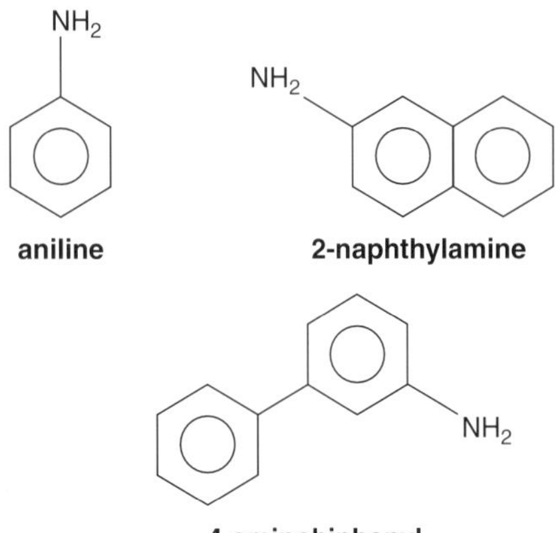

Smokers have a 2–5-fold risk compared to non-smokers, with respect to development of bladder cancer, and subsequent recurrences. Estimates suggest that 25–60% of bladder cancer is caused by smoking.

Occupational exposure to radiation and carcinogens, in particular aromatic hydrocarbons like aniline, is a recognized cause of bladder cancer. Examples of 'at risk' occupations are shown in *Table 9.2*. A latent period of 25–45 years exists between exposure and carcinogenesis.

Other agents reported to cause bladder cancer include the analgesic phenacitin, the cytoxic drug cyclophosphamide and the ova of *Schistosoma haematobium* (bilharziasis).

Pathology and staging

Benign tumours of the bladder, including the inverted papilloma and the nephrogenic adenoma, are uncommon. The vast majority of primary bladder cancers are malignant and epithelial in origin: 90% of bladder cancers are transitional cell carcinomas (TCC), 7% are squamous cell carcinomas (except in areas where schistosomiasis is endemic), 2% are adenocarcinomas and the remainder are sarcomas, arising within the bladder muscle (detrusor). Staging is by the TNM system and may be assessed on clinical (examination, radiology) or histopatho-

Table 9.2:
Occupations associated with TCC

Occupations
Rubber manufacture e.g. tyres or electric cable
Dye manufacture
Fine chemical manufacture e.g. auramine
Retort houses of gas works
Rope and textile manufacturing
Hairdressers
Leather workers
Plumbers
Painters
Drivers exposed to diesel exhaust

Fig. 9.6:
A diagrammatic representation of the T staging of bladder TCC.

T3b
T3a
Pelvic side wall
T2
T1
BLADDER
T4b
Ta
Submucosa
CIS (red patch)
Mucosa (urothelium)
Bladder detrusor muscle
T4a
Prostate
URETHRA

logical criteria. The T staging is illustrated in *Figure 9.6*. Histological grading is divided into 3 groups: well-, moderately, and poorly differentiated, abbreviated to G1, 2 and 3. Locally advanced tumour growth may involve the pelvis, prostate, bowel or obstruct the ureters, while lymphatic or vascular dissemination result in metastases. Common sites include lymph node, lung, liver, and bone.

TCC is caused by all the factors discussed above, except schistosomiasis. They may be single or multiple, and 5% of patients will have a synchronous upper tract TCC. The majority are papillary, exhibiting seven or more layers of well- or moderately differentiated transitional cells covering a fibrovascular core (normal transitional epithelium has approximately 5 cell layers). Papillary TCC (*Fig. 9.7a*) is usually confined to the bladder mucosa (Ta) or submucosa (T1). Solid TCC (*Fig. 9.7b*) is usually poorly differentiated and is frequently invading the detrusor muscle, sometimes locally advanced (T2, 3 or 4). Some TCC has mixed papillary and solid morphology. Ten percent of TCC is flat **carcinoma in-situ** (CIS). This is a poorly differentiated carcinoma, but confined to the epithelium and associated with an intact basement membrane. Half of CIS lesions occur in isolation, appearing as a flat red area; the other half occurring in association with invasive TCC. Genetic alterations reported in TCC include loss of material on chromosome 9 and aberrant expression of the tumour suppressor gene p53 (located on chromosome 17p).

Fig. 9.7:
(a) An endoscopic view of a small papillary TCC of the bladder. (b) An endoscopic view of a small solid TCC of the bladder.

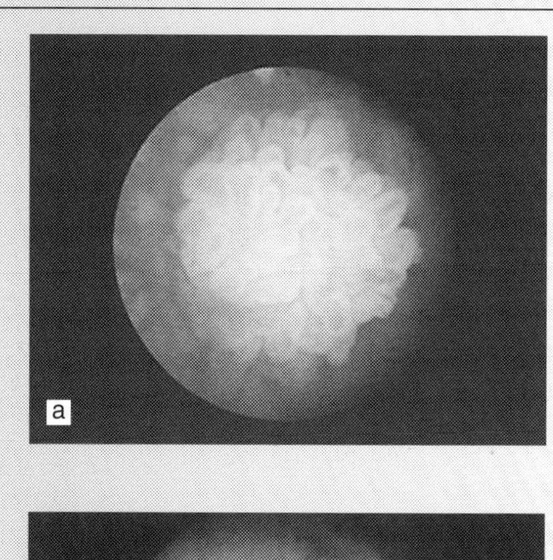

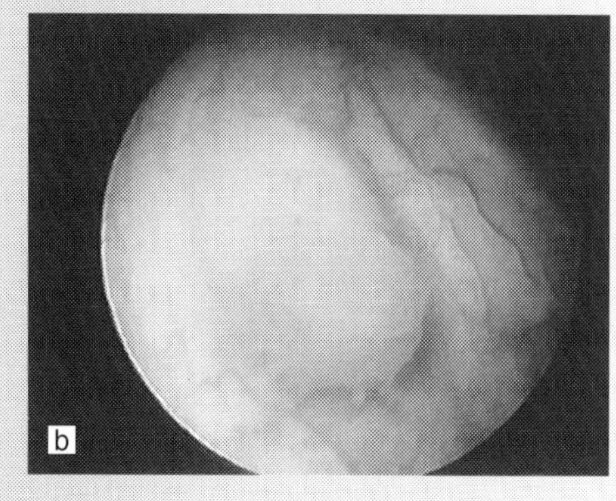

Squamous carcinoma of the bladder is usually solid, muscle-invasive and poorly differentiated. They are caused by chronic inflammation in the bladder, such as those induced by the ova of *Schistosoma haematobium*, stones and indwelling catheters.

Adenocarcinoma of the bladder is rare, usually solid and ulcerative. One third originate in the urachus, the remnant of the allantois; they are located in the dome of the bladder.

Adenocarcinomas are also long-term (20 years or so) sequelae to congenital bladder exstrophy and to bowel implanted into the urinary tract, particularly bladder substitutions after cystectomy. Secondary adenocarcinoma may arise from direct spread of a bowel primary into the bladder.

Presentation

The commonest presenting symptom (80%) is **painless total haematuria**. Pain is unusual, even if the patient has obstructed upper tracts, since the obstruction and renal deterioration arises gradually. The haematuria may be initial or terminal if the lesion is at the bladder neck. Other patients present with **asymptomatic microscopic haematuria**, found on routine urine stick-testing. Up to 16% of females and 4% of males have stick-test haematuria: less than 5% of those below 50 years will have malignancy, while 20% of those >50 years will have a malignancy. Occasionally, a patient will present with urinary tract infections or irritative lower urinary tract symptoms, such as urgency or suprapubic voiding discomfort. This is typical in patients with CIS – so-called 'malignant cystitis'. Although the likelihood of diagnosing bladder cancer in patients under the age of 50 is low, all patients with these presenting features should be investigated. Malignant colovesical fistula is a cause for recurrent urinary tract infections and pneumaturia, though less common than benign causes such as diverticular and inflammatory bowel disease. Examination may reveal pallor, indicating chronic renal impairment or blood loss; abdominal examination is usually unremarkable; rectal examination may reveal a mass if the patient has advanced disease.

Investigations

All patients with microscopic or macroscopic haematuria require investigation of their upper tracts and bladder, provided a urinary tract infection has been excluded or treated. Usually, renal ultrasound, plain X-ray and flexible cystoscopy, performed under local anaesthetic, are first-line investigations. If these fail to find a cause, an IVU and urine cytology are justified. Cytology is frequently (70%) negative in patients with papillary TCC, but more sensitive (80%) in patients with CIS and high-grade TCC. If these are normal, consideration should be given to nephrological disorders that may cause haematuria, such as glomerulonephritis. If there is hydronephrosis in association with a bladder tumour, it must be assumed that the tumour is causing the obstruction to the distal ureter(s) – this tends to be caused by muscle-invasive disease and not superficial cancers.

Staging investigations are reserved for patients with muscle-invasive bladder cancer, since superficial and CIS disease is rarely associated with metastases. These include a pelvic CT scan (*Fig. 9.8*), looking for extravesical tumour extension into perivesical fat, pelvic sidewall or neighbouring structures, a chest radiograph and in certain cases an isotope bone scan (positive in 5–15% of patients with muscle-invasive TCC).

Treatment

If the flexible cystoscopy demonstrates a raised lesion, transurethral resection of bladder tumour (TUR) is undertaken. This is usually done under a general or spinal anaesthetic, so that a bimanual examination may be undertaken after resection to assess for the presence of a residual mass in the bladder. A red patch may be biopsied, since there are numerous non-malignant causes of red patches. These include chronic non-specific cystitis, radiation cystitis and acute cystitis.

Fig. 9.8:
A pelvic CT scan showing a mass deforming the bladder, confirmed to be a muscle-invasive TCC.

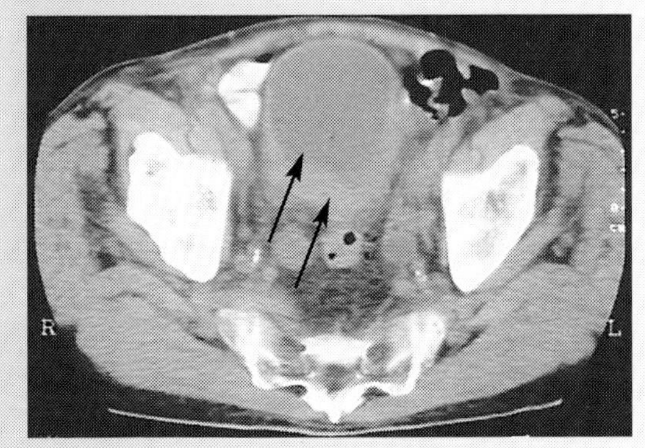

Subsequent treatment or follow-up depends on the histology of the resected lesion, and will be influenced by patient factors such as their age, comorbidity and wishes. *Table 9.3* summarizes current recommendations.

Intravesical chemotherapy (e.g. mitomycin C) is used for G3pT1 tumours and recurrent multifocal TCC. Administered weekly for six weeks, it reduces recurrences by 40%, but has not been shown to prevent progression to muscle invasion and has no impact upon survival. Many patients report transient bladder irritation; occasionally a rash develops on the palms of the hands and treatment must be stopped.

Intravesical BCG (bacille Calmette–Guérin) is also given as a six-week course, for G3pT1 or other multifocal superficial TCC, and for CIS. It reduces recurrences by up to 60%, by acting as an immune adjuvant in upregulating cytokines such as IL-6 and IL-8. It is more toxic than chemotherapy, causing irritative symptoms in nearly all patients and low-grade fever with myalgia in 25%. Rarely, patients develop a high persistent fever, requiring antituberculous therapy.

Radical cystectomy with urinary diversion is the most effective treatment for eradication of curable muscle-invasive TCC, SCC and adenocarcinoma, either primarily or when radiotherapy has failed. It is also used to treat G3pT1 TCC and CIS, refractory to BCG. The entire bladder is excised, along with the prostate in the male and the anterior vaginal wall in the female. Surgical complications include bleeding, thromboembolism, rectal injury and erectile dysfunction. Most cystectomy failures are due to micrometastatic disease in pelvic lymph nodes and soft tissue, undetected by preoperative staging investigations.

Urinary diversion is most commonly attained by formation of an ileal conduit. Here, 15 cm of subterminal ileum is isolated on its mesentery, the ureters are anastomosed to the proximal end and the distal end is brought out as a urostomy. The bowel is re-anastomosed to gain enteral continuity. Complications of ileal conduit are prolonged ileus, urinary leak, enteral leak and stomal problems such as stenosis and parastomal hernia. Alternatives to this form of incontinent diversion include the fashioning of a neobladder from 60 cm of ileum or the right hemicolon. The ureters drain into the neobladder, which fills with urine. This may either be drained via a catheterizable natural tube, such as the appendix or uterine tube – the Mitrofanoff principle – brought out in the right iliac fossa

Table 9.3:
Management of bladder cancer

Histology	Chance of recurrence after TUR	Chance of stage progression	Further treatment	Follow-up
G1/2, pTa/1 TCC	50–70%	10–15%	None	Review cystoscopies, commencing 3 months
G3, pT1 TCC	80%	40%	Intravesical chemotherapy or BCG	Review cystoscopies, commencing 3 months
CIS (carcinoma in-situ)	80%	40%	Intravesical BCG	Cystoscopies and cytology commencing 3 months
pT2/3, N0, M0 TCC, SCC or adenocarcinoma	Usually TUR is incomplete	N/a	Radical cystectomy or radiotherapy	Cystoscopies if bladder is preserved
T4 or metastatic TCC, SCC or adenocarcinoma	N/a	N/a	Systemic chemotherapy; symptom palliation	N/a

giving a continent diversion, or the neobladder may be anastomosed onto the patient's urethra – an orthotopic neobladder – which requires no bags or catheters. Finally, the ureters may be drained into the sigmoid colon – a ureterosigmoidostomy. These more sophisticated forms of urinary diversion are accompanied by complications relating to neobladder leakage, incontinence, stomal stenosis and metabolic abnormalities due to absorption (causing metabolic acidosis) and loss of small bowel (causing vitamin B12 deficiency). Theoretically, adenocarcinomas may develop in neobladder mucosa in the long term due to the carcinogenic bacterial metabolism of urinary nitrosamines.

Radical radiotherapy is a good option for treating muscle-invasive bladder TCC in patients who are elderly, unfit for cystectomy or those who wish to avoid major surgery. The 5-year survival rates are inferior to those of surgery, but the bladder is preserved and many patients do very well. Side-effects include radiation cystitis and proctitis, causing irritative voiding symptoms, diarrhoea and rectal bleeding. These effects usually last only a few months. If disease persists or recurs, salvage cystectomy may still be successful. SCC and adenocarcinoma are less sensitive to radiotherapy than TCC.

Combination chemotherapy is recommended for treatment of metastatic bladder cancer in patients fit enough to tolerate its toxicity. A response rate of 30% is seen.

Palliative measures include radiotherapy for metastatic bone pain, formalin instillation or internal iliac artery ligation for intractable haematuria and ureteric stenting for obstruction. Involvement of a palliative care team can be very helpful to the patient and family.

5-year survival:

pTa /T1 TCC	endoscopic treatment only	95%
G3pT1 TCC	no adjuvant treatment	50%
CIS	no adjuvant treatment	50%
G3pT1 / CIS	adjuvant treatment	90%
G3pT1/CIS	cystectomy	95%
pT2/3 TCC	cystectomy	45–75%
pT2/3 TCC	radiotherapy	20–40%
pT4	radiotherapy	10%
N+ / M+ TCC	radiotherapy/ chemotherapy	5–10%

Prostate cancer

Prostate cancer (PC) is the commonest urological malignancy and the second most common cause of male cancer death. In the UK, there are 19 000 new cases diagnosed each year and 10 000 deaths (1997). Approximately 3% of men die of PC, the overall 5-year survival is 40%. The incidence and mortality are rising in the UK and Europe, while in the USA, there has been a recent fall in mortality. This has fuelled debate about the worthiness of screening.

Risk factors

Age is an important risk factor, the disease being rare below 40 years according to postmortem studies (*Fig. 9.9*) and becoming increasingly common with rising age. This rise is paralleled 20 years earlier by an identified pre-malignant lesion, prostatic intraepithelial neoplasia (PIN). There is a wide **geographic variation** in incidence: the disease is rare in Asia and the Far East, common in Europe and more common in the USA, even including migrants from Asia and Japan. This suggests some environmental influence, such as the Western diet, may be important. **Race** and **family history** are risk factors: black people develop prostate cancer more frequently than whites. The world's highest

Fig. 9.9:
A graph showing the age-related prevalence of prostate cancer and the premalignant lesion PIN in post-mortem studies.

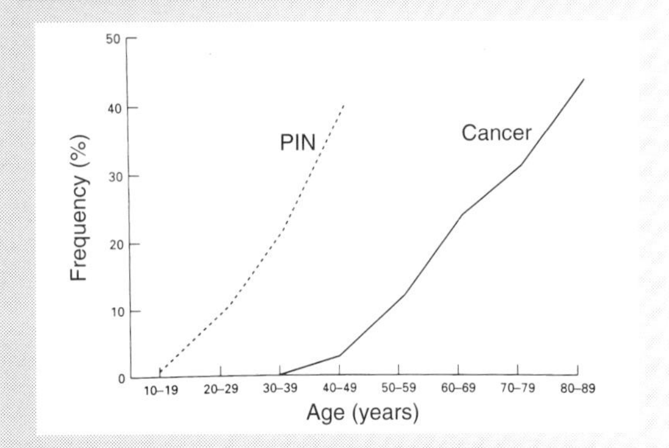

incidence is among US and Caribbean blacks, although there is little data available regarding European and African blacks. PC is hereditary in approximately 5% of cases: a man with one affected first-degree relative (father or brother) has a two-fold risk of developing the disease, while two affected relatives confer a five-fold risk. The race and family history data suggest a constitutional genetic aetiology; indeed, many groups are trying to identify the hereditary prostate cancer gene(s), which may contribute to the much commoner sporadic cancer development. Exposure to **cadmium** has been suggested to raise the risk of PC, but no new data have been forthcoming since the 1960s.

Growth of prostate cancer, like benign prostatic epithelium, is under the promotional influence of testosterone and its potent metabolite, dihydrotestosterone. Removal of these androgens by castration results in programmed cell death (apoptosis) and involution of the prostate. PC is not seen in eunuchs or people with congenital deficiency of 5α-reductase, which converts testosterone to dihydrotestosterone. Oestrogens, including phytooestrogens found in foodstuffs used in Asian and Oriental cuisine, has a similar negative growth effect on PC. Other inhibitors of PC growth include vitamins E and D and the trace element selenium.

Prostate cancer is an interesting disease that has given rise to considerable debate regarding management, particularly screening and the treatment of organ-confined disease. The controversy stems from the disparity between the prevalence of the disease in postmortem studies (*Fig. 9.9*) of up to 40% in octogenerians, the clinical incidence of the disease which affects 10% of all men, and the mortality which is 3% of all men. Part of the explanation for this difference is that PC is a slow-growing disease: the mean cell doubling time is 300 days, so a cancer may take 10 years or more to become clinically apparent (by which point it is likely to be incurable). The challenge for doctors is to identify the fraction of patients with biologically significant disease at an early stage, so that curative treatment can be given without overtreating those who have 'latent' disease. While there are deficiencies in our knowledge of the natural history of PC, it is appreciated that age, comorbidity and biopsy histological grade are important predictors of outcome. Pilot screening studies of asymptomatic men aged 55–70 years have demonstrated a cancer detection rate of 3%: enthusiasts for screening propose that this is the same 3% who would succumb from the disease.

Pathology and staging

The vast majority of primary PC is adenocarcinoma. Primary TCC of the urethra and prostatic ducts is uncommon, though the prostate may be involved by a locally advanced (T4) bladder TCC. Rhabdomyosarcoma is an occasional and aggressive stromal tumour, more commonly seen in children than adults. Secondary deposits are rare in the prostate.

Most (75%) PC arises in the peripheral zones (PZ) of the prostate. A few PCs arise anteriorly or within the transition zones, so are impalpable on digital rectal examination (DRE). Macroscopically, they tend to be hard and white, though a soft mucin-producing variety exists. Microscopically, adenocarcinoma is graded 1 to 5 according to its gland-forming differentiation by the **Gleason scoring system** (*Fig. 9.10*). Most PC is multifocal, so an allowance is made for this in the grading, by adding the two dominant grades to give a sum-score between 2 and 10. In practice, 75% of PC is graded 5, 6 or 7, 10% are graded 2, 3 or 4 and 15% are graded 8, 9 or 10.

Prostatic intra-epithelial neoplasia (PIN) is equivalent to carcinoma in-situ, without breach of the epithelial basement membrane (*Fig. 9.11*). Often seen in biopsies alone or in association with PC. Studies have shown that if PIN is seen in isolation, repeat biopsies reveal invasive PC in 50% of cases. It appears to be a premalignant lesion, found in young men in postmortem studies (*Fig. 9.9*).

Genetically, PC is complex, generally exhibiting numerous abnormalities, increasing with stage and grade. Frequent changes include somatic loss of alleles on chromosomes 8, 16 and 18, inactivation of tumour suppressor genes pTEN and p53 and activation of c-myc and bcl-2 proto-oncogenes.

PC is staged by the TNM system (*Fig. 9.12*). PC, like most carcinomas, spreads by local extension beyond the flimsy prostatic capsule, or metastasizes via the lymphatic or venous systems. Common

Fig. 9.10:
A diagrammatic representation of the Gleason grading system for prostate cancer. The grade depends on the structure of the prostatic glands and their relationship to the stromal smooth muscle.

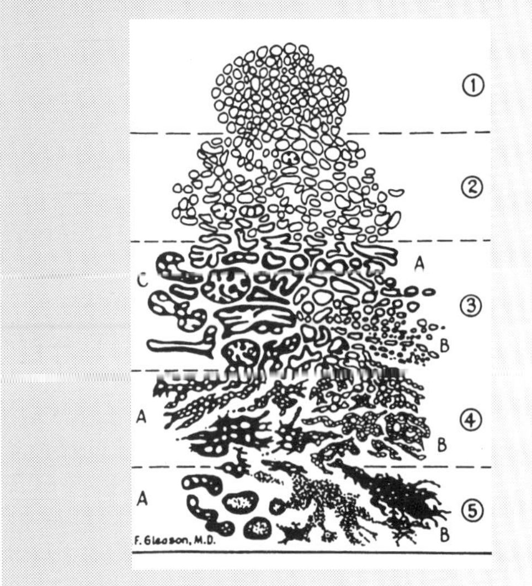

sites of metastasis include the axial skeleton, the long bones, lymph nodes, lung and liver. In short, T1/2 N0M0 represents organ-confined disease, potentially curable; T3/T4 N0M0 represents locally advanced disease, rarely curable and T1–4, N1 or M1 represents advanced disease, currently incurable.

Fig. 9.11:
A histological slide (H&E) showing PIN in a prostatic duct. The cells are irregular and piled up, forming a cribriform pattern.

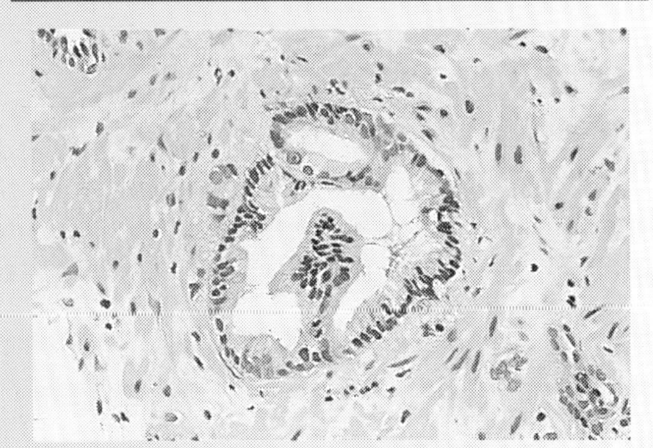

Presentation

Lower urinary tract symptoms. While frequently caused by co-existent benign prostatic hyperplasia, most men present with lower urinary tract symptoms (LUTS) due to bladder outflow obstruction (BOO). PC is all too often incurable at presentation because it is not organ-confined. Features in the history suggestive of PC include rapidly progressive LUTS, predominantly irritative in nature. The concurrent appearance of bone pain, malaise or weight loss may suggest metastatic disease. General examination may demonstrate cachexia, clinical anaemia, lymphadenopathy or oedema of a lower limb, suggestive of pelvic lymphatic obstruction. Abdominal examination may reveal a palpable bladder if BOO is causing chronic retention, or rarely hepatomegaly. Locally advanced PC rarely causes priapism by infiltration of the corpora cavernosa. DRE may be normal or reveal abnormality such as asymmetry, nodule, local extension or fixed craggy mass. A clinical T stage should be assigned after DRE. Haematuria is an occasional presenting symptom.

Haematospermia is an occasional presenting symptom of PC. Often self-limiting and undiagnosed, this symptom should be investigated if it is persistent, particularly in men of 50 years or older.

Backache is a common presentation of 'occult' metastatic PC. The axial skeleton, particularly the lumbar spine and pelvis, and the long bones are the most common sites for distant metastasis. The pain is usually of fairly recent onset, worsening, continuous and requires analgesia. This differs from the more common musculoskeletal pains that tend to be chronic, slowly progressive and related to time of day or movement. A spinal metastasis may **compress the spinal cord** within the vertebral canal, resulting in an acute neurological deficit, motor or sensory. Any man who develops acute neurological lower limb symptoms or 'goes off his legs' should have a careful neurological examination and a DRE.

Fig. 9.12:
A diagrammatic representation of the T stage of prostatic carcinoma.

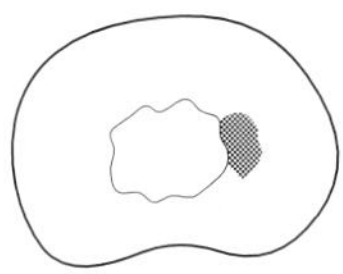

T1a – Carcinoma
in ≤5% of TURP specimen,
non-palpable

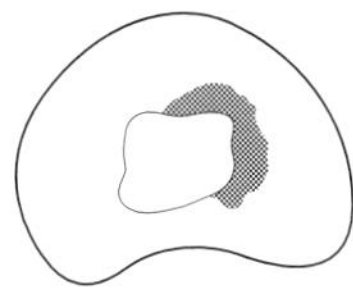

T1b – Carcinoma
in ≥5% of TURP specimen,
non-palpable

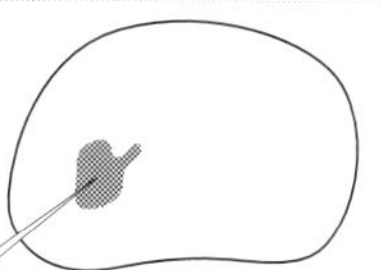

T1c – Carcinoma
in needle biopsies,
non-palpable

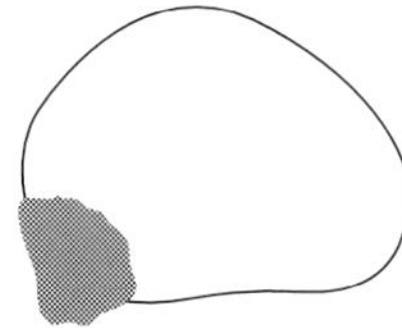

T2a – Carcinoma
of one side,
palpable

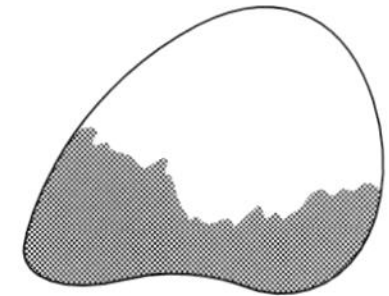

T2b – Carcinoma
of both sides,
palpable

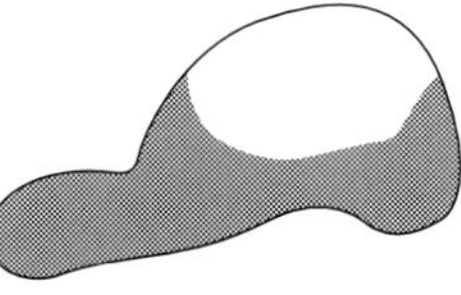

T3a – Carcinoma
growing beyond the capsule
into periprostatic fat

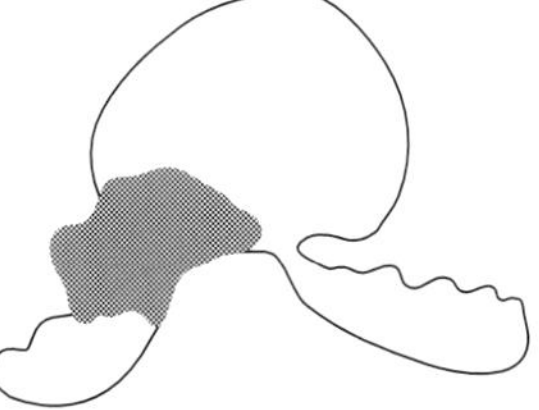

T3b – Carcinoma
growing into the
seminal vesicle

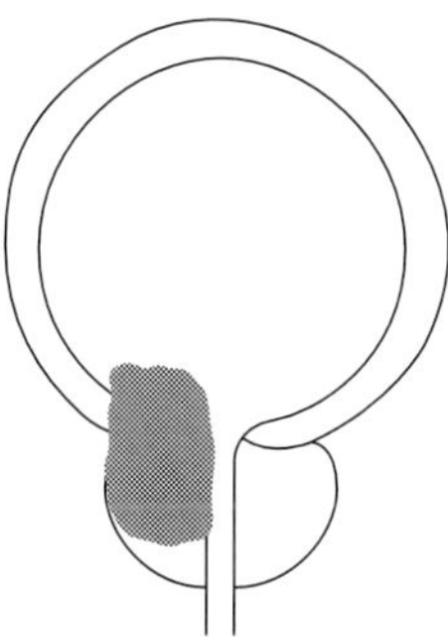

T4 – Carcinoma
growing up into bladder, ureter,
down into root of penis or
posteriorly around rectum

Asymptomatic men are increasingly presenting, either requesting or having had screening tests. These tests are the serum prostate specific antigen (PSA), with or without a DRE. There is currently no national screening programme in the UK, but many private health insurers are including PSA in their 'well-man screening clinic' investigations. Patients should be counselled before these tests are carried out. In the USA, where annual screening with PSA and DRE is recommended to all men aged 50–75 years, most men now present with organ-confined PC.

Chest symptoms, jaundice, anaemia, malaise and weight loss are occasional presenting symptoms, indicative of advanced disease. Often, the diagnosis is delayed because symptoms are non-specific.

The DRE. Since most PCs arise in the peripheral, posterior part of the prostate, they should be palpable by DRE. An abnormal DRE is defined by asymmetry, a nodule, or a fixed craggy mass. Approximately 50% of abnormal DREs are associated with PC on biopsy, the remainder being benign hyperplasia, prostatic calculi, chronic prostatitis, or post-radiotherapy change. The fact that an abnormal DRE in the presence of a normal PSA carries a 30% chance of predicting PC (see *Table 9.4*) rules out the suggestion by some that the DRE could be abandoned.

Table 9.4:
The chance of PC on biopsies

PSA (ng ml^{-1})	0.1–1.0	1.1–2.5	2.6–4.0	4–10	>10
DRE normal	1%	5%	15%	25%	>50%
DRE abnormal	5%	15%	30%	45%	>75%

Table 9.5:
Conditions excluding PC which cause falsely elevated PSA

Cause of PSA	Minor elevation <1.0 ng ml^{-1}	Major elevation 1.0–100 ng ml^{-1}
Benign hyperplasia	√	√
Urinary infection		√
Acute or chronic prostatitis		√
Retention/ catheterization		√
Biopsy, TURP		√
Ejaculation, DRE	√	

Investigations

Prostate specific antigen (PSA). PSA is a glycoprotein enzyme produced by the prostate. Its function is to liquefy the ejaculate, enabling fertilization. Large amounts are secreted into the semen, and small quantities are found in the urine and blood. PSA does not appear to perform any function in the blood, where 75% is bound to plasma proteins and metabolized in the liver while 25% is free and excreted in the urine. The half-life of PSA is 2 days. The normal range for the serum PSA assay is usually <4.0 ng ml^{-1}. The predictive values of PSA and DRE for % chance of finding PC in biopsies are shown in *Table 9.4*. Causes of a false positive PSA are shown in *Table 9.5*.

In the presence of infection or instrumentation, PSA should be requested at least 28 days after the event, to avoid unnecessary concern by doctor and patient. Ideally, PSA should not be requested within 2 days of ejaculation or DRE, but in practice it makes negligible difference to the result and the management of the patient.

The specificity of PSA can be increased by applying the **age-specific normal range** (95th centile), shown in *Table 9.6*, to help decide whether to recommend biopsies. Although widely used, this remains controversial. Consideration should also be given to prostate volume, since large benign prostates are the most common cause of mildly elevated PSA.

Measurement of the **free-to-total PSA ratio** is helpful in deciding whether to repeat biopsies in a patient with a total PSA of 4–10 ng ml^{-1}, who has had previous benign biopsies. This is because the ratio is lower in men with PC than in men with benign hyperplasia. While overall a man with a normal DRE and a PSA of 4–10 ng ml^{-1} has a 25%

Table 9.6:
The age-adjusted normal range for PSA

Age range	Normal PSA range ($ng\,ml^{-1}$)
All ages	<4.0
40–49	<2.5
50–59	<3.5
60–69	<4.5
>70	<6.5

risk of PC, this risk rises to 60% if his ratio is 10% and falls to 10% if his ratio is 25% or greater.

A PSA that is rising by >0.75 ng ml^{-1} per year over two or more years is suggestive of the presence of PC. This is called PSA velocity.

Serum creatinine electrolytes and renal ultrasound are indicated to exclude obstruction to the kidneys, either by ureteric obstruction due to locally advanced PC or BOO.

Transrectal ultrasonography with prostatic biopsies is currently the most common diagnostic modality, the other being at TURP. It is generally indicated in the presence of an abnormal DRE and/or an elevated PSA. Exceptions include very elderly men with massively elevated PSA or abnormal DRE, or those in whom a TURP is indicated for BOO or severe LUTS. Repeat biopsies are indicated if isolated PIN is seen on previous biopsies or if there is ongoing concern due to rising PSA or abnormal DRE. The procedure is undertaken on an outpatient basis without anaesthetic. It takes 10 minutes: most patients find it uncomfortable, but not painful. Broad-spectrum antimicrobials are given before and after, since there is a <1% risk of septicaemia. Usually, 6–12 Tru-cut needle biopsies are taken in a systematic fashion, including any palpable or sonographic target lesion. It is important also that the patient appreciates that negative biopsies do not exclude the possibility of PC, and that a positive result will not necessarily result in the recommendation of immediate treatment.

An **isotope bone scan** is reasonably sensitive in detecting metastatic disease, which show as 'hot spots' (Chapter 2, *Fig. 2.4*). If the PSA is <20, only 2% of bone scans will demonstrate metastases. False-positive results occur around arthritic joints and in bones affected by Paget's disease. Plain radiographs may be helpful, although the characteristic sclerotic (bone-forming) metastases of PC may still be confused with Paget's disease. Magnetic resonance imaging (MRI) of the bone marrow is more sensitive than isotope bone scanning, though more expensive (Chapter 2, *Fig. 2.5*).

Pelvic MRI is often helpful in demonstrating local extension of PC (*Fig. 9.13*) and in detection of lymph node enlargement indicative of metastatic PC.

A **chest X-ray** occasionally demonstrates pulmonary lesions, mediastinal lymphadenopathy or lymphangitis carcinomatosa.

Treatment

Stage T1a PC is clinically unsuspected prior to TURP. It is usually low-grade and low-volume. Long-term progression to advanced disease occurs in 15% of patients. There is little dispute that this stage of PC can be managed with observation, a 6-monthly DRE and PSA, treating only if there is evidence of disease progression.

Fig. 9.13:
A transverse pelvic MRI showing a prostate cancer (the dark area in the centre of the scan) with invasion of the bright-signalling seminal vesicles, hence staged T3b. Top is posterior.

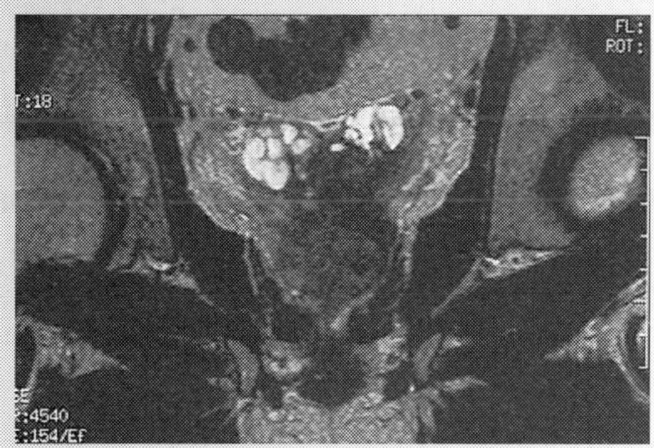

Stage T1b, T1c and T2 PC demands considerable thought and discussion, particularly if the patient is under 70 years and may live more than 10 years. Accurate assessment of the likelihood of non-organ confined disease can be obtained using the staging investigations discussed above, and nomograms based on the clinical T stage, PSA and biopsy grade. These nomograms are known as Partin's tables, after their author. It is important to appreciate that 50% of men with PC and a PSA >10 ng ml^{-1} will have advanced disease. The likelihood of metastatic disease and death due to PC after 10–15 years of observation can be considered using published data, according to biopsy grade. *Table 9.7* summarizes these data.

(a) **Observation**: a respectable option for genuine low-grade PC (in which the results of the more aggressive treatments described below are no better), for men who are >75 years or for those with significant medical comorbidity such that their life expectancy is judged to be <10 years. If the disease progresses during follow-up, palliative treatment, such as **androgen ablation therapy** (AAT), is recommended.

(b) **Radical external beam radiotherapy (EBRT)**: a 6-week course of daily treatments amounting to a dose of 60 Gray. A non-invasive attempt to cure PC, sometimes accompanied by temporary AAT. Reasonable long-term results, with few side-effects, except 30–50% develop erectile dysfunction (ED). Salvage prostatectomy in cases which are failing is seldom an option.

Table 9.7:
15-year natural history of localized PC managed with observation

Biopsy grade	% risk of metastasis	% risk of death	Lost years of life
2 to 4	19	4–7	<1
5	42	6–11	4
6	42	18–30	4
7	42	42–70	5
8–10	66	60–87	6–8

(c) **Brachytherapy**: ultrasound-guided implantation of radioactive seeds, usually I^{125}, into the prostate (*Fig. 9.14*). Minimally invasive 'day-case' procedure requiring general anaesthetic. Currently popular, having failed in the 1970s prior to transrectal ultrasonography. Good long-term results from one US institution. Poor outcome in patients with BOO or larger prostates. Few complications except up to 25% risk of urinary retention, 5% incontinence and 50% ED. Salvage EBRT is an option in patients who have rising PSA if local recurrence is suspected.

(d) **Radical prostatectomy**: the current gold standard. Excellent long-term results in well-selected patients, particularly those with BOO. A major operation, it involves transabdominal or transperineal excision of the prostate and seminal vesicles (*Fig. 9.15*), with reconstruction of the bladder neck and vesico-urethral anastomosis. Complications are those of major surgery (bleeding, thromboembolism), 70% ED, 5% incontinence after 6 months and 10% urethral stricture. Overall, 30% have a detectable PSA by 10 years follow-up. These patients can be offered salvage EBRT if local recurrence is suspected. The time to development of metastatic disease after having a detectable PSA averages 8 years.

Fig. 9.14:
An X-ray showing placement of the radiopaque I^{125} seeds during prostate brachytherapy. The tip of the transrectal ultrasound probe is seen at the bottom of the film.

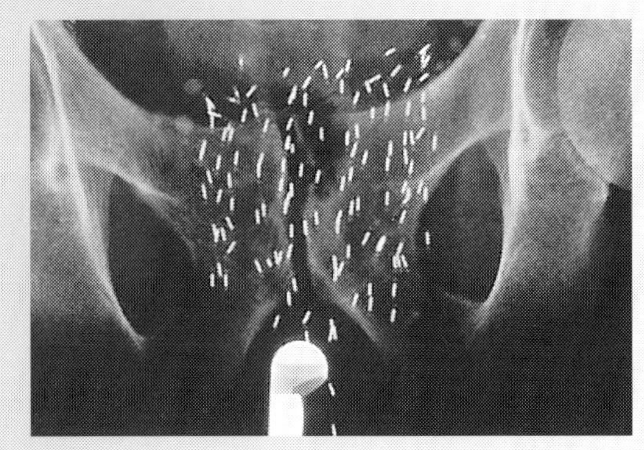

Fig. 9.15:
A radical prostatectomy specimen.

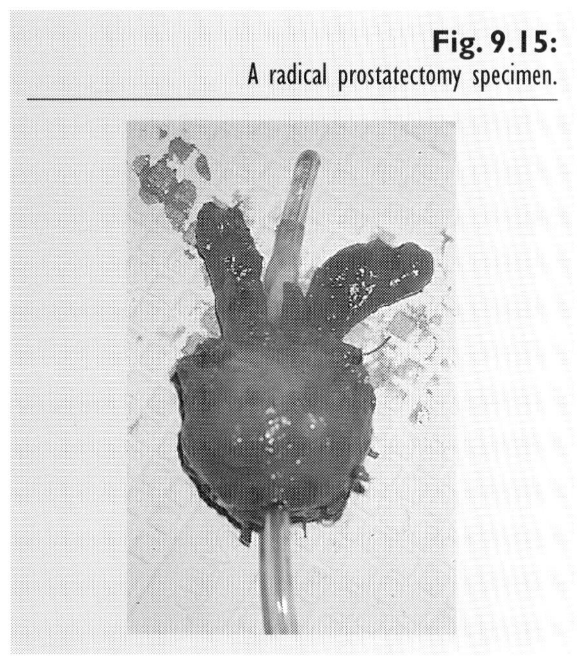

Which option is taken may be decided after lengthy discussions and more than one opinion may be sought by the patient. Unfortunately, a prospective British trial of prostatectomy vs. radiotherapy vs. observation failed to recruit and was abandoned in 1995. Most treatment failures are due to micrometastatic disease in pelvic lymph nodes and bone, undetected by preoperative staging investigations. Local recurrence is also possible, particularly after radiotherapy.

Stage T3/4 N0M0 PC is treated palliatively since it is incurable. Having said this, respectable 5-year results are obtained using radiotherapy in combination with 2 years of adjuvant AAT. The alternative is to recommend long-term AAT. A comparison of these two treatments is the subject of a current MRC trial. In addition to these treatments, complications of the disease such as BOO, ureteric obstruction or rectal stenosis may require expeditious surgical management.

Stage N1/M1 (metastatic) PC requires systemic palliative treatment. The 5-year survival is 25%. The first-line approach is AAT, which will produce a response in 75% of patients for a mean time of 18 months. There has been debate on whether AAT should be commenced prior to symptoms of metastatic disease: results of an MRC trial suggest it should, since it may prevent catastrophes like spinal cord compression and may improve survival. Bilateral orchidectomy or depot injections of luteinizing hormone-releasing hormone (LHRH) analogues such as goserelin acetate are equally effective forms of AAT. Oral antiandrogens (for example, bicalut-amide) may be added to block peripheral androgen receptors to the effects of adrenal androgens. Most trials have failed to demonstrate benefit with this manoeuvre, called maximal androgen blockade. Non-responders and patients relapsing on AAT may respond to further manipulations, including the addition withdrawal of antiandrogens, or mild chemotherapy regimens, for example, intravenous mitoxantrone. Again, emergent procedures may be required, including radiotherapy for bone pain or spinal cord compression, internal fixation of a pathological fracture, TURP for BOO, or ureteric stenting for hydronephrosis with renal failure. The involvement of palliative care physicians and Macmillan nursing is often very helpful in the terminal phase of the illness.

Screening for PC. Screening men aged 50–70 years with PSA and DRE may reduce the significant mortality and morbidity caused by PC. It is an acceptable and relatively inexpensive test. However, because of the low specificity of the test, many men would suffer unnecessary anxiety and biopsies. Some men with PC may be overtreated and the treatment options have their own morbidity and are expensive. Currently there are no plans for a PC screening programme in the UK, although the results of a huge European randomized trial are awaited.

Neoplasia of the ureter and retroperitoneum

Ureteric tumours are uncommon, accounting for 1% of urinary tract neoplasia, while retroperitoneal tumours are rare. The majority are malignant, TCC and liposarcoma are the most common types, respectively. Staging is by the TNM system. Benign ureteric fibroepithelial polyps can cause diagnostic uncertainty. Ureteric TCC shares aetiological factors with TCC of the renal pelvis and bladder, the major being cigarette smoke (see page 96).

Presentation

Ureteric tumours may present with painless haematuria or loin pain. Retroperitoneal sarcomas present with symptoms including abdominal or back pain, weight loss, a swollen leg, urinary or bowel symptoms. Because of these non-specific symptoms, diagnosis is frequently made late. Examination is often unremarkable, although an abdominal mass or lower limb oedema may be present with retroperitoneal sarcoma.

Investigations

Ultrasound will reveal hydronephrosis if the ureteric or retroperitoneal tumour is causing ureteric obstruction. IVU, retrograde or antegrade ureterography will demonstrate the site of the lesion, revealing a filling defect or 'apple core' ureteric stricture in the case of a ureteric tumour, or a tapering stricture if the compression is extrinsic (*Fig. 9.16*). Urine cytology may be positive with ureteric TCC. Abdominal CT scan is the best investigation for demonstrating retroperitoneal sarcomas. Chest radiography is essential to exclude metastases.

Fig. 9.16:
An antegrade ureterogram showing a long filling defect in an obstructed distal ureter. This patient had a history of bladder TCC but had not experienced loin pain.

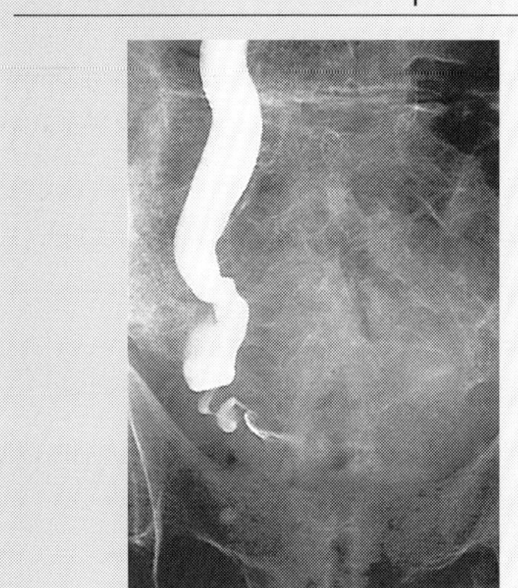

Treatment

Ureteric TCC: for lesions in the upper and middle thirds of the ureter, nephroureterectomy is indicated, in the presence of a functioning contralateral kidney. For lower third tumours, it may be possible to perform a local excision and primary anastomosis, to reimplant the ureter into a bladder flap or elongated bladder, or into the contralateral ureter (a transureteroureterostomy).

Retroperitoneal sarcomas: surgical removal via a transperitoneal approach. Incomplete excision is a problem since the tumour often extends microscopically beyond its pseudocapsule. Adjuvant radiotherapy is often recommended.

Follow-up cystoscopies and IVU are required for TCC; follow-up CT scans are required for retroperitoneal sarcomas.

5-year survival:

Ureteric TCC: 90% if excision is complete.

Retroperitoneal sarcomas: 50%.

Testicular cancer

Primary testicular cancer (TC) is the most common solid cancer in men aged 20–45. It is also considered the most curable cancer, with 1380 new cases reported but only 77 deaths per year in the UK (1997). It is increasing in incidence, reported to affect 7 per 100 000 men. Public health campaigns encouraging testicular self-examination (TSE) for young men are ongoing. Metastases to the testis are rare, notably from the prostate.

Risk factors

Age: the commonest affected age group is 20–45 years, with germ cell tumours. Teratomas are more common in adults aged 20–35, while seminomas are more common in the 35–45 age-group. Rarely, infants and boys below 10 years and men older than 60 years can develop yolk sac tumours and lymphomas respectively.

Race: white people are four times more likely to develop TC than black people.

Cryptorchidism: 10% of TC occur in undescended testes, the risk increased by 3–14 times compared to men with normally descended testes. There are reports of a 5% risk of in situ malignant change in the normally descended contralateral testis.

Human immunodeficiency virus (HIV): patients infected with the HIV virus are developing germ cell tumours more frequently than expected.

Genetic factors may play a role, but a defined familial inheritance pattern is not apparent.

Pathology and staging

Ninety per cent of testicular tumours are malignant germ cell tumours, 8% are stromal and 1% are metastatic. Seminomas appear pale and homogeneous (*Fig. 9.17*), while teratomas are heterogeneous and sometimes contain bizarre tissues such as cartilage or hair. *Table 9.8* shows the classification of testicular tumours.

TC is staged using the TNM system. TC spreads by local extension into the epididymis, spermatic cord and rarely the scrotal wall. Lymphatic spread occurs via the testicular vessels, initially to the para-aortic nodes. Blood-borne metastasis to the lungs, liver and bones occurs.

Presentation

The majority of patients present with a painless lump in the scrotum. Occasionally acute scrotal pain may occur, due to intratumoral haemorrhage, causing diagnostic confusion with testicular torsion or orchitis. Symptoms suggestive of advanced disease include weight loss, chest symptoms and bone pain. Physical examination may reveal cachexia, supraclavicular lymphadenopathy, chest signs, hepatomegaly, lower limb oedema or abdominal mass, all suggestive of metastatic disease. Examin-ation of the genitalia will reveal a hard non-tender irregular mass in the testis, or replacing the testis. Rarely, a hydrocele may be present. The spermatic cord may be normal or thickened. Gynaecomastia is rare.

Fig. 9.17: A radical orchidectomy specimen, sectioned to reveal a homogeneous tumour, consistent with the appearance of a seminoma.

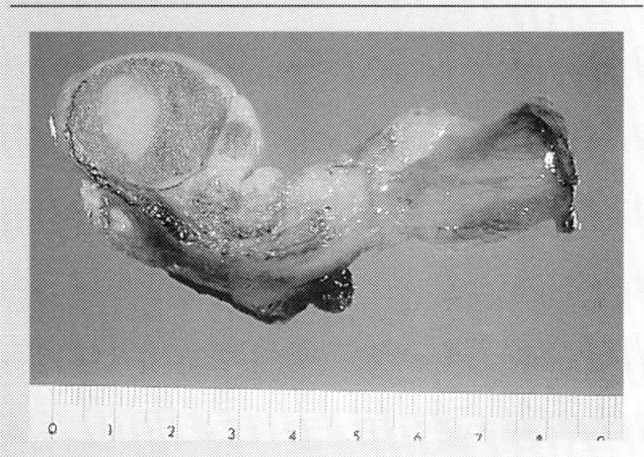

Table 9.8: The classification of testicular tumours

Germ cell tumours	Stromal tumours (10% malignant)	Other tumours
Seminoma	Leydig cell	Epidermoid cyst (benign)
Teratoma: differentiated intermediate undifferentiated	Sertoli cell	Adenomatoid tumour
Mixed seminoma/teratoma	Mixed	Adenocarcinoma of the rete testis
Yolk sac tumour		Carcinoid
Choriocarcinoma		Lymphoma
		Metastatic

Investigations

Ultrasound will confirm that the palpable lesion is within the testis, distorting its normally regular outline and internal echo pattern.

Serum markers:

(a) Alpha-fetoprotein (AFP) is expressed and secreted into the bloodstream by 50–70% of teratomas and yolk sac tumours.

(b) Human chorionic gonadotrophin (hCG) is expressed and secreted into the bloodstream by 40% of teratomas and 15% of seminomas.

(c) Lactate dehydrogenase (LDH) is expressed and secreted into the bloodstream by 10–20% of seminomas.

These markers are measured at presentation, after radical orchidectomy and during follow-up to assess response to treatment and residual disease.

Abdominal and chest CT scans are usually obtained after histological diagnosis is made, for staging purposes.

Treatment

The primary treatment for all testicular tumours is **radical orchidectomy**. This involves excision of the testis, epididymis and cord, with their coverings, through a groin incision. The cord is transfixed and divided before the testis is manipulated into the wound, preventing inadvertent metastasis. A silicone prosthesis may be inserted at the time, or at a later date. This treatment is curative in approximately 80% of patients.

Further treatment depends upon the histology and staging CT scans. Benign tumours need no further follow-up. Patients with malignant tumours are usually seen by the clinical oncologist. If the disease appears to be confined to the surgical specimen and postoperative serum markers are normal, surveillance with periodic markers and CT scans is recommended. If staging or markers suggest systemic disease, systemic **combination chemotherapy** is recommended. Various regimes of chemotherapy exist, for example bleomycin, etoposide and cisplatin. **Radiotherapy** to enlarged para-aortic nodes is an alternative, in the case of metastatic seminoma.

For residual para-aortic node enlargement after chemotherapy, **retroperitoneal lymph node dissection** may be curative. This surgery is invasive, carrying a high risk of ejaculatory and erectile dysfunction.

5-year survival:

90–95%, following radical orchidectomy with adjuvant chemotherapy or radiotherapy. Liver and brain metastases carry a poor prognosis.

Penile cancer

Penile cancer is uncommon, representing 1% of male cancers, most occurring in elderly men. Approximately 400 new cases and 100 deaths are reported annually in the UK.

Risk factors

Age: penile cancer is rare below the age of 40.

Premalignant lesions: various lesions, usually appearing on the glans penis as chronic painless red or pale patches, are premalignant. These include leukoplakia, erythroplasia of Queyrat, and the Buschke-Löwenstein tumour.

A foreskin (prepuce): penile cancer is rare in men circumcised at a young age. It is virtually non-existent in Israel. It is thought that chronic irritation with smegma and balanitis in men who are unhygienic is contributory.

Human papilloma virus (HPV) wart infection, especially with types 16, 18 and 21, is implicated.

Pathology and staging

Squamous cell carcinoma is the commonest penile cancer (*Fig. 9.18*). Occasionally basal cell carcinoma occurs. It starts on the glans or foreskin, preceded by carcinoma in-situ, and grows locally beneath the foreskin before invading the corpora cavernosa, urethra and eventually the perineum, pelvis and prostate. Metastasis to inguinal and subsequently pelvic lymph nodes is slow, and blood-borne metastasis to lungs and liver is rare. Staging is by the TNM system.

Presentation

A hard painless lump on the glans penis is the most common presentation. Frequently the lump is surprisingly large, but has gone unnoticed, or ignored, beneath the foreskin. Sometimes the lesion will

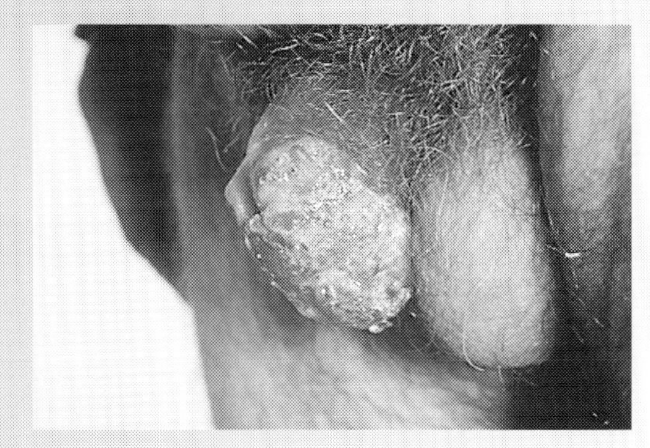

Fig. 9.18: A photograph of a squamous carcinoma of the glans penis. The foreskin has been destroyed by the tumour.

give rise to a bloody discharge on the patient's underwear, so may be confused with haematuria. A chronic red or pale patch on the glans is a cause for concern. Examination of the penis may reveal an obvious tumour, hard and non-tender, beneath the foreskin. In more advanced cases, the foreskin and glans are replaced by fungating tumour, growing to involve the shaft, scrotum and even the perineum (*Fig. 9.18*). If there is a patch on the glans, note should be made of its colour, size and surface features. If the glans and foreskin are normal, penile cancer is most unlikely. Occasionally, a patient may be alarmed by a subcutaneous lump on the penile shaft. This is often accompanied by some penile deviation at erection. Examination may reveal a smooth non-tender plaque on one of the corpora cavernosa. This is the benign fibrosing lesion of Peyronie's disease and the patient may be reassured that no biopsy is required.

The inguinal lymph nodes may be palpably enlarged, either due to metastasis or reaction to infection of the primary tumour.

Investigations

In many cases, the diagnosis is not in doubt. A **chest X-ray** is usually obtained. If there is diagnostic doubt, a **penile biopsy** is indicated. This may necessitate a circumcision. This also applies to chronic red or pale patches on the glans, unresponsive to antibacterial or antifungal creams or if they are growing larger, raised or bleeding.

Treatment

The first-line treatment of penile cancer, regardless of the inguinal node status, is surgery. Occasionally, **circumcision with wide excision** of any glanular lesion is adequate. Usually however, **partial or total penile amputation** is required, depending on the extent of the tumour. If the patient has distant metastases, surgery is offered to palliate symptoms. Partial amputation is preferable, provided a 2 cm margin of palpably normal shaft can be obtained. The patient may need to sit to pass urine following this surgery, which is frequently curative. Total amputation involves excision of the scrotum and its contents, with formation of a perineal urethrostomy. Local recurrence occurs in 10%, if the excision margin is not clear.

Carcinoma in-situ lesions may be successfully treated with laser ablation, topical chemotherapy (5-fluorouracil cream), plastic surgery or radiotherapy.

Lymphadenopathy is treated with a six-week course of broad-spectrum **antimicrobials**, after the primary tumour has been removed. The nodes become clinically insignificant in 50% of patients, who may then be observed periodically. In those with persistent inguinal lymphadenopathy, provided staging chest radiography and abdomino-pelvic CT are normal, **bilateral inguinal lymph node dissection** may be considered, since this may be curative. However, this is major surgery, with a high incidence of complications including lymphocele development and wound breakdown. It is not suitable for elderly, unfit men. An alternative treatment is **radiotherapy** to palpable nodes.

Systemic single-agent **chemotherapy** is recommended for distant metastatic disease.

5-year survival:

Node-negative SCC	65–90%
Inguinal node metastases	30%
Metastatic SCC	<10%

Carcinoma of the urethra

Primary urethral cancer is rare, occurring in elderly patients, more commonly in women. Direct spread from tumour in the bladder or prostate is more common. Urethral stricture and sexually-transmitted disease have been implicated as risk factors.

Pathology and staging

Tumours are mostly squamous cell carcinomas (75%), though 10% are TCC and the remainder are adenocarcinomas. Urethral cancer metastasizes to the pelvic nodes, and to the inguinal nodes in 30% of patients. Staging is by the TNM system.

Presentation

Presentation is often late and many patients have metastatic disease at presentation. Patients may present with painless haematuria, typically initial or terminal, or a bloody discharge. Obstructive voiding symptoms or perineal pain are less common complaints. Periurethral abscess or urethrocutaneous fistula are rare presentations. Examination may reveal a palpable mass at the female urethral meatus, or along the course of the male urethra. Inguinal lymphadenopathy, chest signs and hepatomegaly may suggest metastatic disease.

Investigations

Cystoscopy, biopsy and bimanual examination under anaesthesia will obtain a diagnosis and local clinical staging.

Chest radiography and abdomino-pelvic CT scan will enable distant staging.

Treatment

For localized urethral cancer, **radical surgery or radiotherapy** are the options. Results are better with surgery. Postoperative incontinence due to disruption of the external sphincter mechanism is minimal unless the bladder neck is involved. For locally advanced disease, a combination of preoperative radiotherapy and surgery is recommended. For metastatic disease, chemotherapy is recommended.

5-year survival:	
Surgery: anterior urethra	50%
Surgery: posterior urethra:	15%
Radiotherapy:	34%
Radiotherapy and surgery:	55%

Scrotal cancer

A rare disease, originally described to occur in Victorian chimney sweeps, by Percival Pott. It was thus the first cancer to be associated with an occupation. It is a squamous cell carcinoma, which presents as a painless lump or ulcer on the anterior or posterior (therefore not obvious if the patient is lying or sitting) scrotal wall. Local inguinal lymphadenopathy may suggest metastasis or reaction to infection. Treatment of a mass or ulcer on the scrotum in wide local excision. Antimicrobials are administered for six weeks if there is lymphadenopathy, then re-evaluated. Inguinal lymphadenectomy is considered if lymphadenopathy persists, with adjuvant chemotherapy.

Key points

- **All** patients with microscopic or macroscopic haematuria in the absence of infection require urological investigation.
- **All** solid renal masses require excision and not percutaneous biopsy.
- Smoking predisposes to transitional cell carcinoma and renal cell carcinoma.
- In the absence of screening, **most** patients with newly diagnosed prostate cancer are incurable.
- More men die **with** prostate cancer than **of** prostate cancer.
- **Most** clinically organ-confined prostate cancer requires treatment in men whose life expectancy exceeds 10 years.
- Serum PSA is elevated by many benign conditions including hyperplasia and infection.
- **All** solid testicular masses require excision of the testis and spermatic cord.
- Testicular cancer carries an excellent prognosis following treatment.

Cases

1. A 58-year-old woman presents with a single episode of painless total haematuria. She is a smoker and has a past history of a pulmonary embolus, apparently related to hormone replacement therapy, which she has now stopped taking. Examination was unremarkable. Her general practitioner had arranged a renal ultrasound which demonstrated a 5 cm right renal mass.
   (a) Which other investigations are indicated?
   (b) Which treatment is indicated?
   (c) Which thromboembolism prophylaxis should be recommended?
   (d) What follow-up is required?

2. A 54-year-old fit man reported troublesome urinary frequency and a dribbling flow. The prostate was enlarged and clinically benign on DRE. His urologist carried out a transurethral resection of the prostate (TURP). The pathology returns, unexpectedly, showing 'well-differentiated' carcinoma in 50% of the resected specimen. His PSA at follow-up was 5.3.
   (a) What stage is this PC?
   (b) What further information is required?
   (c) What are the treatment options?

3. A 22-year-old man presented with a painless hard lump in his right testicle, which his girlfriend noticed the previous week. He had lost half a stone over the previous 3 months, attributed to a recent period detained at Her Majesty's pleasure. Ultrasound confirmed a testicular tumour.
   (a) Which immediate investigations are requested?
   (b) Which treatment is indicated?
   (c) Which further investigations are indicated?
   (d) What further treatment is recommended in the case of metastatic teratoma?

Answers

1. (a) This patient has a renal tumour. She should have CT scans of chest and abdomen, to exclude metastatic disease and renal vein invasion and to check function of the contralateral kidney by administration of intravenous contrast. However, she should also have a cystoscopy, since there may be a synchronous TCC (remember, she is a smoker). Her CT scans revealed the solid mass in the right upper renal pole, with no other abnormality. The cystoscopy revealed a papillary bladder tumour.
   (b) A transurethral resection of the bladder tumour and a radical nephrectomy.
   (c) Lower limb compression stockings should be applied and either intermittent pneumatic calf compression or subcutaneous heparin prescribed until the patient is fully mobile.
   (d) This depends on the pathology reports. In fact, her renal tumour was an oncocytoma, which requires no follow-up. The bladder tumour was a G2pTa TCC, which requires regular review cystoscopies and occasional IVUs.

2. (a) T1b.
   (b) This patient still has PC and is likely to progress long term. The pathology of the resected specimen should be reviewed by a pathologist familiar with the Gleason system, since truly low-grade disease is quite uncommon (10% chance). Upon review, a Gleason sum of 3 + 3 = 6 was assigned. Contemplating aggressive treatment, he had a bone scan and a pelvic MRI scan, which demonstrated no evidence of extraprostatic disease.

(c) The options are observation, radical radiotherapy or radical prostatectomy. Brachytherapy is contraindicated because of the high risk of incontinence. After discussion, he chose surgery, from which he made an excellent recovery. PC was observed close to the surgical margin at the prostatic apex, but his PSA 6 weeks postoperatively was undetectable. Nevertheless, he remains at risk of relapse, so must be followed-up long-term.

3. (a) Serum AFP, hCG and LDH for baseline information.
   (b) A radical orchidectomy through the groin.
   (c) A CT scan of chest and abdomen, which unfortunately revealed para-aortic lymphadenopathy and 'cannon-ball' lung metastases.
   (d) Combination platinum-based chemotherapy. A retroperitoneal lymph node dissection is not offered, since there was complete resolution of all metastatic disease on follow-up CT scans.

Further Reading

Albertsen P.C., Hanley J.A., Gleason D.F. and Barry M.J. Competing risk analysis of men aged 55 to 74 years at diagnosis, managed conservatively for localised prostate cancer. *JAMA* 1998; **280**: 975–980.

Catalona W.J., Smith D.S., Ratliff T.L. and Basler J.W. Detection of organ-confined prostate cancer is increased through PSA-based screening. *JAMA* 1993; **270**: 948–954.

Chodak G.W., Thisted R.A., Gerber G.S., Johansson J.E., Adolfsson J., Jones G.W., Chisholm G.D., Moskovitz B., Livne P.M. and Warner J. (1994) Results of conservative management of clinically localized prostate cancer. *N Engl J Med* **330**: 242–248.

Gillenwater J., Grayhack J.T., Howards S.S. and Duckett J.W. (1996). *Adult and Paediatric Urology*. Third ed. Mosby, St. Louis.

Partin A.W., Kattan M.W., Subong E.N., Walsh P.C., Wonjo K.J., Oesterling J.E., Scardino P.T. and Pearson J.D. (1997) Combination of PSA, clinical stage and Gleason score to predict pathological stage of localized prostate cancer. A multi-institutional update. *JAMA* **277**: 1445–1451.

Resnick M.D. and Novick A.C. (1995). *Urology Secrets*. Hanley & Belfus, Philadelphia.

U.I.C.C. (1997). *TNM Classification of Malignant Tumours*. Fifth ed. Wiley-Liss, New York.

CHAPTER 10

Andrology and benign genital conditions

Male infertility

One in 10 couples fail to conceive a child after a year of unprotected intercourse. Persons presenting after this time warrant evaluation. One-third of cases of infertility result from male factors, one-third from female factors and one-third from mixed contributory factors. Hence, ideally both male and female should be evaluated simultaneously. The causes of male infertility are shown in *Table 10.1*.

Clinical assessment of the infertile male

History

First establish the duration, frequency and timing of unprotected intercourse and ensure that libido, erection, penetration and ejaculation are normal. Previous medical/surgical and drug histories may establish a likely cause. Previous pregnancies, either with the present or a previous partner, are indicative that the infertility is acquired. A family history of cystic fibrosis may point to congenital absence of the vasa.

Table 10.1: Differential diagnosis of male infertility

Treatable causes	Potentially treatable causes	Untreatable causes
Varicocele	Idiopathic	Bilateral anorchia
Ejaculatory and sexual dysfunction: phimosis, hypospadias	Congenital or acquired vasal absence or obstruction	Primary testicular failure: germ cell aplasia
Infection: prostatitis	Cryptorchidism	Secondary testicular failure: bilateral torsions, trauma or infection: mumps, tuberculosis
Endocrine: hyperprolactinaemia, hypogonadotrophic hypogonadism	Drugs: cimetidine, marijuana, alcohol, nitrofurantoin, hormones, steroids	Chronic disease e.g. renal or liver failure, diabetes mellitus
Immunological: antisperm antibodies	Surgery or trauma causing vasal injury e.g. childhood hernia repair	Chemotherapy/radiotherapy (patients having these treatments should be advised to store semen frozen)
	Occupation/recreational: hot environments e.g. driving, saunas, tight trousers	

Examination should include urinalysis (for evidence of infection), general inspection for signs of chronic disease, abnormal body hair or gynaecomastia. Examination of the external genitalia is made to assess the presence, size and consistency of the testes in the scrotum. Absent testes indicate cryptorchidism and small soft testes suggest testicular failure. Bulky epididymes may indicate vasal obstruction. The presence of both vasa is confirmed by palpation of structures in each spermatic cord that feel like string. A careful inspection is made for the presence of a varicocele **by standing the patient up**. A large varicocele is obvious with the patient lying, while a moderate one may only be detectable with the patient standing, classically described to feel like a bag of worms. A small varicocele may only be detectable by listening with a Doppler probe applied to the scrotal wall and asking the patient to cough. Examining the penis, a phimosis or hypospadias may be present which could impair ejaculation. Finally, a DRE is performed to assess for prostatic tenderness, which indicates prostatitis.

Investigations

Semen analysis: At least two fresh ejaculates obtained 48 hours apart should be examined. Normal values are shown in *Table 10.2*

A 'stress pattern' of **oligospermia** with reduced motility and increased abnormal forms is often associated with varicocele, drugs, smoking and elevated temperatures. **Azospermia** indicates testicular failure or obstruction.

Table 10.2: Normal semen analysis

Volume	1.5–5 ml
Sperm density	>20 million ml^{-1}
Motility	>60%
Abnormal forms	<40%
Leucocytes	none

Hormonal evaluation: serum LH, FSH, prolactin and testosterone

- ↓FSH+LH: hypogonadotrophic hypogonadism
- ↑FSH: testicular failure; germinal epithelial damage associated with azospermia and oligospermia depicting significant and irreversible germ cell damage.
- ↑Prolactin: possible pituitary tumour

Chromosomal studies: a buccal smear is indicated if Klinefelter's or Turner's syndrome are suspected.

Immunological studies: agglutination tests for antisperm antibodies, reserved for patients with previous history of torsion, injury, vasectomy.

Testicular biopsy with vasography: for patients with suspected testicular failure or vasal obstruction.

Transrectal ultrasonography (TRUS) may reveal signs of prostatitis or calculi obstructing the ejaculatory ducts.

Treatment

General

The stress pattern can be improved by cessation of smoking, drugs or modification of alcohol consumption, lifestyle changes such as wearing loose trousers and boxer shorts and taking cool baths or showers. Intercourse should be no more than twice per week, timing with ovulation if possible.

Medical

Immunological. Prednisolone can be used against antisperm antibodies, but there is a risk of side-effects including avascular necrosis of the head of the femur.

Prostatitis. In young patients, whether organisms are cultured or not, a six-week course of ciprofloxacin and doxycycline will treat most bacterial or chlamydial prostatitis.

Surgical

Varicocele repair. A varicocele is present in 40% of infertile men, yet only 15% of all young men. Repair by ligation of the veins in the groin or trans-femoral radiological embolization (*Figs. 10.1a and b*)

Fig. 10.1:
(a) A transfemoral left renal venogram showing flow of contrast down a dilated testicular vein with no functioning venous valve; (b) following embolization using titanium coils, preventing downward passage of contrast.

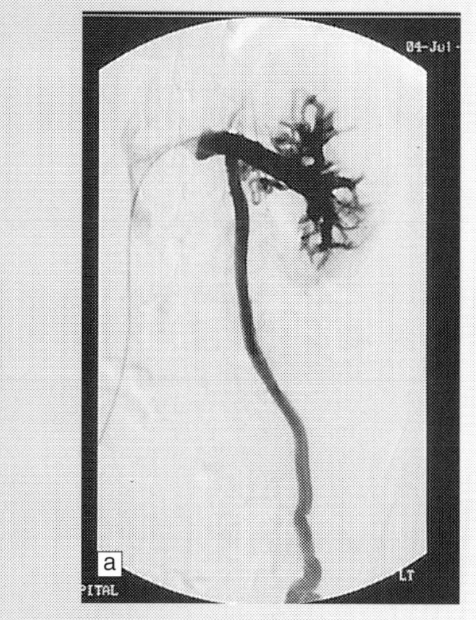

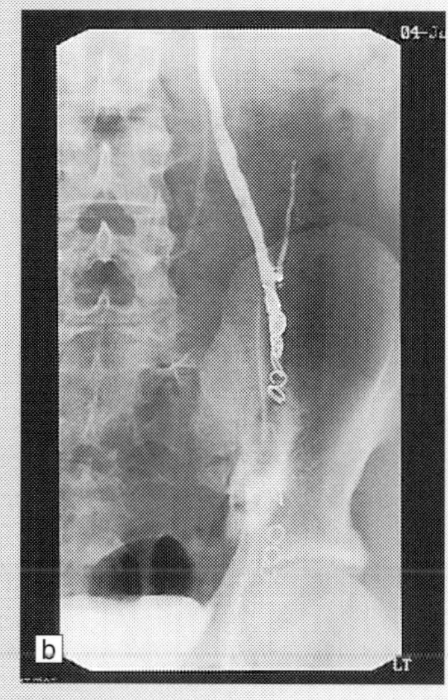

improves the semen analysis in 70% of patients with the stress pattern. 40% achieve pregnancy. It is believed this works by cooling the affected testis.

Vasovasostomy in patients with localized vasal obstruction or previous vasectomy: 50% achieve pregnancy overall.

Circumcision, hypospadias surgery, electroejaculation or voided sperm washing may all be helpful to patients with ejaculatory disorders.

Assisted fertilization techniques. 30% achieve a pregnancy, often multiple. Techniques are expensive and generally available only on a private basis. MESA or TESA (microsurgical epididymal sperm aspiration or testicular sperm aspiration) are undertaken if sperms exist in the epididymis or testis. In men with testicular failure, successful conceptions have been reported with testicular aspiration and assisted conception techniques, but most couples need to consider artificial insemination by donor or adoption. Acquired sperms can be used for assisted uterine implantation or IVF (in-vitro fertilization) techniques, including subzonal sperm injection (SUZI) and intracytoplasmic sperm injection (ICSI).

Erectile dysfunction

Physiology of normal erection

Visual or tactile stimulation of the thalamic autonomic erection centre results in impulses being transmitted via the cavernosal branches of the pudendal nerves, containing fibres from T12–L2 and S2–S4, to nerve endings in the cavernosal artery smooth muscle. This stimulates the release of neurotransmitters, including nitric oxide and prostaglandins. This causes the activation of guanylate and adenylate cyclase, increasing local concentrations of cGMP and cAMP. These neurotransmitters cause relaxation of the smooth muscle and the cavernosal arteries dilate, increasing blood flow into the cavernosal sinuses. As they fill, the sinuses compress the subtunical venules, resulting in reduced venous outflow from the corpora cavernosa (*Fig. 10.2a*). The corpora become engorged, increasing their length and girth and becoming rigid. Reduction in the release of neurotransmitters coupled with the metabolism of cGMP and cAMP by phosphodiesterases reduces inflow, increases venous outflow and detumescence occurs (*Fig. 10.2b*).

Fig. 10.2:
The physiology of penile erection: (a) development; (b) resolution.

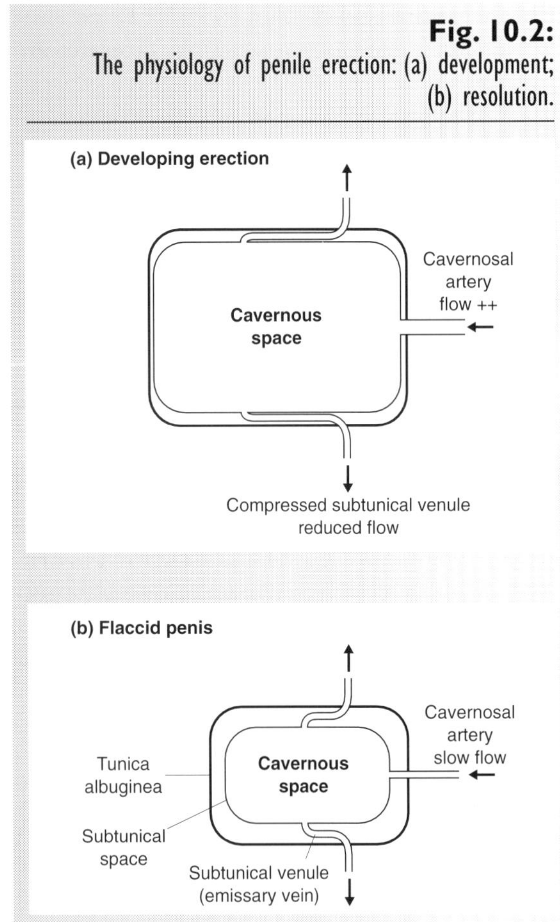

Erectile dysfunction

Erectile dysfunction (ED) is defined as the failure to obtain or maintain an erection satisfactory for sexual intercourse. Contrast this with **premature ejaculation**, defined as the uncontrolled ejaculation before or shortly after the penetration, and **retrograde ejaculation**, defined as ejaculatory backflow due to incompetence of the bladder neck. ED is said to affect 5% of healthy 40 year olds and 15% of 70 year olds, excluding those with clear organic causal factors. Two basic types of ED exist: psychogenic and organic. The causes of the two types are shown in *Table 10.3*.

Clinical assessment of the male with ED

History

Ensure that ED is truly the presenting complaint and establish the duration of the complaint and any life-event to which its onset was related. A good way to distinguish psychogenic from organic ED is by determining whether the patient ever wakes with an erection (nocturnal penile tumescence), which indicates a psychogenic aetiology. The past medical and drug histories may reveal the aetiology. A social history is important, in terms of ascertaining detail of relationships, smoking and alcohol consumption.

Table 10.3:
Causes of ED

Psychogenic ED	Organic ED
Stress	Chronic disease: renal, liver, diabetes, atheroma
Performance anxiety	Trauma: pelvic surgery, prostatectomy, pelvic fracture
Previous sexual abuse	Prostate cancer
Previous sexual relationship problems/dysfunction	Peyronie's disease
Mental state disorders	Neurogenic: multiple sclerosis, spinal injury
	Drugs: antihypertensives, LH/RH analogues, antidepressants, cimetidine, alcohol
	Hypogonadism: pituitary or gonadal
	Infection: prostatitis

Examination

This should begin with a general inspection for signs of hypogonadism such as altered body hair and physique. Examine the external genitalia and carry out DRE as described above. In addition, examine the peripheral pulses to detect any generalized large vessel disease. Finally, a stick-test urinalysis may reveal glucose, indicating diabetes mellitus (sometimes previously undiagnosed), or leucocytes, indicating infection.

Investigations

If there are symptoms and signs to suggest hypogonadism, a serum testosterone and prolactin are indicated. There are a variety of sophisticated tests that measure penile blood-flow velocity using Doppler sonography, intracavernosal pressures (cavernosometry) and mapping of venous outflow (cavernosography). However, these investigations are academic in the vast majority of patients with ED, so are not undertaken.

Treatment

General measures

Patients are advised to stop smoking and reduce alcohol consumption. Alteration of the patient's drugs may help. Psychogenic ED is in theory best treated by appropriate psychosexual counselling. In practice, such counsellors are scarce and tend to work privately.

Pharmacotherapy

Oral phosphodiesterase type 5 inhibitor: sildenafil (Viagra) maintains high concentrations of cGMP in the cavernosal smooth muscle, facilitating maintenance of erection. Sexual stimulation and nerve conduction is required. Overall, 70% of men with ED achieve a satisfactory erection within 45 minutes of ingestion. Similar results are obtained regardless of aetiology, except only 40% of patients with pelvic nerve injuries are satisfied. There is some concern about prescribing sildenafil to men with a history of cardiac disease, but a definite contraindication is the concurrent use of nitrates for angina, hypertension or cardiac failure. There have been reports of hypotension and fatal arrhythmias in such circumstances. Currently, only patients with diabetes, neurological illnesses, prostate cancer, previous pelvic surgery and 'severe distress' may obtain sildenafil using an NHS prescription.

Prostaglandin E1 (PGE1): alprostadil is currently available as an intracorporeal injection or as a urethral pellet. These work by increasing the concentrations of cAMP in the cavernosal smooth muscle, by providing substrate for adenylate cyclase. Because neurotransmitters are not required, PGE1 produces an erection rapidly in 80% of patients, without the need for sexual stimulation. A greater proportion of men with neurogenic ED will also respond to PGE1. However, a significant number of patients report pain at the injection sites or in the urethra. There is a 1% risk of priapism developing.

Premature ejaculation is often effectively treated with clomipramine (Anafranil). If retrograde ejaculation is the complaint, ephedrine or phenylpropylamine can tighten the bladder neck sufficiently for antegrade ejaculation to occur.

Physical treatments for ED

Vacuum/constriction pump: this device, costing £100–200, is placed over the penis and a pump produces a vacuum. A constricting rubber ring is placed around the base of the penile shaft to maintain rigidity. No needles are required, however the erection looks a rather unhealthy colour and hangs at an unnatural angle, so it is not very popular.

Penile prosthesis: prostheses are implanted down the corpora in place of the erectile tissue. They are either solid (rigid or malleable) or inflatable, via a pump and reservoir placed in the scrotum. They are particularly suitable for men with Peyronie's disease associated with ED, since the Nesbit straightening procedure is often unsatisfactory in these circumstances. Five percent become infected, particularly in diabetics, and must be removed. They are expensive.

Revascularization procedures: seldom undertaken. Occasionally recommended for a trauma patient, in whom arteriography has demonstrated an operable discontinuity in one or both internal pudendal arteries. Venous ligation procedures for 'leaks' often fail as new venous channels open.

Benign genital conditions

Priapism, **penile fracture**, **testicular torsion** and **torsion of the appendix testis** are discussed in Chapter 3. **Phimosis** and **paraphimosis** are discussed in Chapter 11. **Epididymitis** and **orchitis** are discussed in Chapter 7.

Peyronie's disease

Peyronie's disease is a fibromatosis of unknown aetiology, affecting focal areas of the tunica albuginea of the corpora cavernosa. Described in 1743, it can be a sexually crippling condition, affecting men in their fifth and sixth decades.

Symptoms usually start with development of focal penile pain on erection. Gradually, deviation of the erection progresses, sometimes until penetration and intercourse are impossible, or too painful for the patient and his partner. The pain lasts 6–9 months, subsiding to leave the deviation which progresses no further. Twenty percent of patients also complain of ED, with distal penile flaccidity. Examination reveals a fibrous non-tender plaque on one or both corpora. The patient may confirm that this causes the deviation during erection. There should be no sinister features about the plaque and no inguinal lymphadenopathy. It is sometimes helpful to obtain a photograph of the erection, or simulate an erection by a test injection of PGE1, to assess the deviation objectively, before offering treatment. A total of 15% of patients also have Dupuytren's contracture.

Treatment should not be offered until the disease has stabilized, when the pain resolves. Then, if intercourse is unsatisfactory, surgery is the gold standard treatment. Various non-surgical treatments have been advocated, including vitamin E and interferon injections, with limited success. The Nesbit procedure involves excising ellipses of tunica and closing the defects, opposite the plaque (*Fig. 10.3*). By producing artificial erections per-operatively, the penis can be straightened in erection. A circumcision is mandatory and the patient must be warned that the surgery will produce about 1 cm of shortening.

If ED is a problem in Peyronie's disease, a Nesbit procedure is best done with insertion of penile prostheses (see above), since the combination of shortening and ED is an unsatisfactory outcome.

Fig. 10.3: The Nesbit procedure for the correction of penile deformity caused by Peyronie's disease.

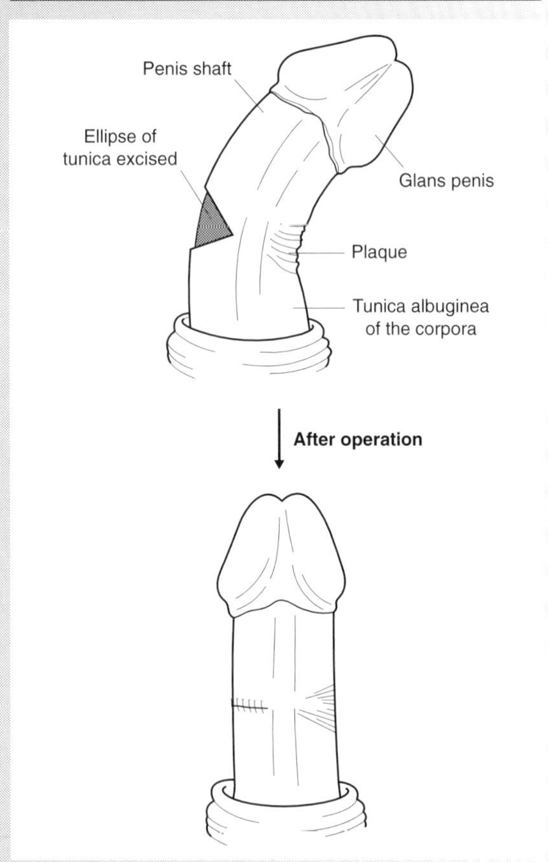

Redrawn from *Essential Urology 1st Edn.*, Bullock *et al.*, Fig. 21.5, 1989, by permission of the publisher Churchill Livingstone.

Inguinoscrotal hernia

This is seen in young boys and older men. In boys, it is caused by congenital persistence of a patent processus vaginalis (PPV) and is associated with undescended testis. It may contain peritoneal contents or just fluid if the neck is narrow. In men, it is an indirect inguinal hernia, which may contain peritoneal contents. In 10% of patients, the sac also contains bladder and even distal ureter, the sliding hernia 'en glissade'. Presentation is usually with a painless lump in the scrotum, which may disappear when the patient if lying. Occasionally the hernia may contain strangulated peritoneal contents, presenting acutely with a painful lump in the groin and scrotum. Examination may reveal a swelling only when the patient stands and it is not possible to 'get above' a hernia on palpation. It may or may not be reducible when the patient is lying. The swelling may transilluminate if the sac contains only fluid. Surgical repair, with ligation of the hernia sac at the level of the internal inguinal ring, is indicated.

Hydrocele

Aetiology

A common cause of scrotal swelling in all age-groups. Hydroceles may be primary or rarely secondary to chronic epididymal infection (e.g. filariasis, tuberculosis), trauma or testicular tumour. The aetiology of primary hydrocele is unknown, but amber-coloured fluid containing cholesterol crystals collects inside the tunica vaginalis, surrounding the testis, epididymis and distal cord (*Fig. 10.4a*).

Presentation

Usually with a longstanding painless scrotal swelling, although they can cause discomfort if large (*Fig. 10.4b*). The swelling is always present, gradually increasing in size, unless the hydrocele communicates with the peritoneal cavity, as in the case of boys with PPV. It may be bilateral. Clinically, hydroceles vary considerably in size, but should not cause a swelling in the groin. The swelling may obscure the contralateral testis and even the penis. With the patient standing, it should be possible to 'get above' the swelling and palpate the spermatic cord; if not, it is probably a hernia. It is not possible to reduce the swelling, unless there is a PPV. The swelling may be lax or tense, the latter obscuring palpation of the ipsilateral testis and epididymis. It is smooth, fluctuant and transilluminates. If associated with trauma, it may not transilluminate because it contains blood or haematoma – a **haematocele**. Regional inguinal lymph nodes are normal.

Fig. 10.4:
(a) Diagram showing the anatomy of a hydrocele; (b) a Zanzibari man with large hydrocele, secondary to filarial lymphatic obstruction.

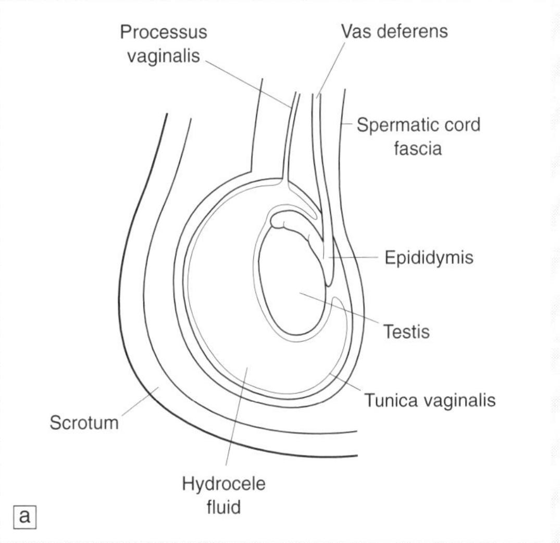

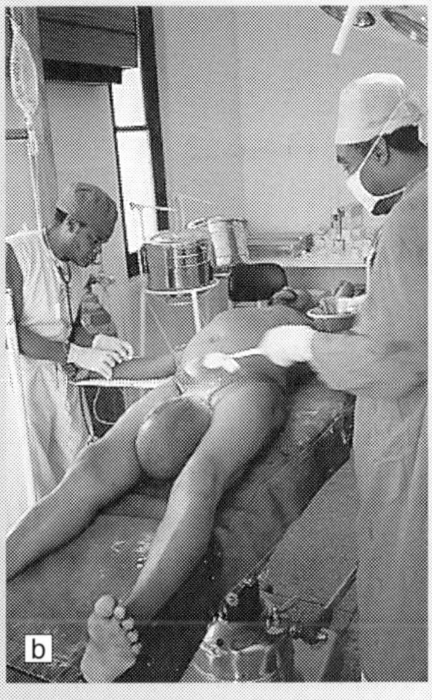

Investigations

Scrotal ultrasound will exclude a testicular tumour in young men with a short history of the swelling.

Treatment

Infants and children are usually managed by paediatric surgeons, by exploring the spermatic cord in the groin to ligate a PPV if present. In adults, hydroceles require treatment only if they are causing discomfort or forcing the patient to purchase larger trousers! They may be **aspirated** percutaneously under local anaesthetic, but this should be undertaken under sterile conditions to avoid introducing infection. Unfortunately, the hydrocele will often re-accumulate; this may be prevented by introduction of a **sclerosant** after the sac is aspirated to dryness. This technique is reserved for elderly, unfit men. Repair by opening the tunica vaginalis in the scrotum is the gold standard treatment. The tunica may be plicated or turned 'inside-out' by wrapping it around the epididymis. Either way, the hydrocele will not recur.

Epididymal cyst

Another common cause of scrotal swelling in all age groups, they cause discomfort more often than hydroceles. These cysts, for they are often multiple, are thought to arise from congenital diverticulae of the epididymal tubules. They may be bilateral and are benign, since malignancy in the epididymis is rare. The cysts usually contain clear watery fluid, although they may contain sperm and the fluid is milky (a **spermatocele**). Epididymal cysts are usually tense, spherical, transilluminable and sometimes tender. They are differentiated from hydroceles by the separate palpation of the testis and cord, unless they are large and multiple which can cause confusion. The swelling is typically above and behind the testis. It should be possible to get above the swelling with the patient standing. Treatment is surgical excision if the cyst is causing discomfort. The patient should be warned that they can 'recur' in a different place. Aspiration is not recommended because they recur. Sclerosant injection is painful.

Varicocele (see also Male infertility)

This is a varicose dilatation of the pampiniform venous plexus running with the spermatic cord. It is present in 15% of all men. It is commoner on the left, where the testicular vein drains vertically into the renal vein. On the right, the testicular vein drains non-vertically into the inferior vena cava. They are classified into: grade 1, subclinical and detectable using Doppler ultrasound; grade 2, palpable when the patient is standing; grade 3, visible as a scrotal swelling and palpable when the patient is lying.

Presentation

Most varicoceles are asymptomatic. Grade 2 and 3 varicoceles can **ache**, typically after prolonged standing or towards the end of the day. The sudden appearance of a left varicocele in an older man should raise suspicion of an underlying **renal cancer** with vein invasion. A total of 40% of infertile men have a varicocele, usually asymptomatic. Grade 2 and 3 varicoceles feel like a bag of worms when the patient is standing. The testis is often smaller than that of the unaffected side.

Investigation

Ultrasound will confirm the diagnosis if necessary. Renal ultrasound is indicated in older patients.

Treatment

Repair by ligation of the veins in the groin or transfemoral radiological embolization are the recommended treatments for symptomatic varicoceles, or those thought to be causing infertility.

Vasectomy

This procedure is commonly performed by general practitioners under local anaesthesia via two short scrotal incisions. It is associated with certain problems about which the patient and his partner must be counselled pre-operatively. They must be aware that:

(a) vasectomy may be irreversible;
(b) there is a 1 in 8000 risk of spontaneous late recanalization of the vas, potentially resulting in unexpected conception;
(c) sperms may appear in the ejaculate up to 3 months after vasectomy, so alternative contraception must be used until two semen analyses have shown no sperm;
(d) if sperms persist in the ejaculate, the procedure may need to be repeated;

(e) there is a small chance of wound infection and scrotal haematoma postoperatively;
(f) there is a 1% risk of chronic scrotal pain, possibly due to extravasation of sperms and chronic inflammation.

Despite all this, vasectomy remains a popular method of contraception. General anaesthesia is advisable if the patient is very anxious, obese or has had previous scrotal or groin surgery.

Vasectomy reversal (vaso-vasostomy)

This procedure is advised for men who wish to be fertile again after vasectomy. It is more successful if the vasectomy was performed <5 years earlier. It is not available on the NHS, but is less costly and more successful than IVF. Preoperatively, the two ends of the cut vas on each side are identified (they feel like pieces of string). If they cannot be palpated, they may be too widely separated to be anastamosed. Complications include haematoma (10%) and failure to achieve sperms in the ejaculate (30%). The chance of pregancy is 40–70% depending on time elapse since vasectomy.

Key points

- If a varicocele is detected during the investigation of male infertility, it should be treated either by embolization or ligation.
- The finding of small soft testes and a grossly elevated serum FSH indicates testicular failure. Successful conceptions have been reported with testicular aspiration and assisted conception techniques, but most couples need to consider artificial insemination by donor or adoption.
- The best way to distinguish psychogenic from organic ED is by determining whether the patient ever wakes with an erection (nocturnal penile tumescence). If so, his ED is psychogenic.
- Sildenafil (Viagra) is currently the first-line treatment for organic and most psychogenic erectile dysfunctions. It is contra-indicated if the patient is prescribed nitrates.
- Peyronie's disease causes a lump on the tunica of the corpus cavernosum, which can cause alarm to patients. When the diagnosis is made, the patient should be reassured that there is no cancer and no need for a biopsy.
- The only way to exclude testicular torsion as a cause of acute scrotal pain if in doubt is to explore the scrotum under anaesthetic. The finding of testicular torsion should prompt bilateral orchidopexy.

Cases

1. A fit 35-year-old man has been trying for a baby with his wife for 15 months. She is the same age and has had two children by a previous marriage. His semen analyses have shown sperm densities of 8 and 10 million ml^{-1}, 30% motility and 60% abnormal forms.
   (a) What do we call this semen analysis result?
   (b) Which features are important in the history?
   (c) What should be sought on examination?

2. A 42-year-old judge with no past medical history reported a gradual failure of his ability to sustain his erections, despite a good libido. He is a non-smoker and there has been no change to his alcohol consumption for years. He reports some urinary frequency.
   (a) Which other points are relevant in the history?
   (b) Which signs are sought on examination?
   (c) Which investigation is vital?
   (d) What treatment will be offered?

Answers

1. (a) This is oligospermia, with a stress pattern.
   (b) We can assume that this couple's infertility is due to male factors. Knowledge of his lifestyle and smoking, alcohol and drug habits is important. Apparently he takes cool showers, wears boxer shorts and has no habits.
   (c) The external genitalia should be examined lying and standing, with a Doppler ultrasound probe at hand. Particular care is taken to detect a varicocele. If identified, it should be treated. He was referred for varicocele embolization. Two months later, his sperm density was 25 million ml^{-1}.

2. (a) A judge may suffer stress at work, so psychogenic ED is a possibility. Does he get good nocturnal erections? Apparently not, so his ED is likely to be organic.
   (b) Signs of hypogonadism (loss of body hair and small testes) are unlikely to be observed because his libido is normal. Loss of peripheral pulses is unlikely in a non-smoker of his age. No signs may be observed.
   (c) A urinalysis, looking for evidence of infection and diabetes mellitus. His stick-test contained +++ glucose. Subsequently, his fasting blood glucose was 12 mmol l^{-1} and he was referred to a diabetologist for advice. His urinary frequency was due to polyuria; it improved after his diabetes was controlled.
   (d) Sildenafil (Viagra) was prescribed. The standard 50 mg dose was ineffective, but fortunately 100 mg enabled a satisfactory erection.

Further Reading

Gillenwater J., Grayhack J.T., Howards S.S. and Duckett J.W. (1996). *Adult and Paediatric Urology*. Third ed. Mosby, St. Louis.

Resnick M.D. and Novick A.C. (1995). *Urology Secrets*. Hanley & Belfus, Philadelphia.

CHAPTER 11

Paediatric urology

Urological problems in children and adults are sometimes related to congenital anomalies of the genito-urinary (GU) tract. In this chapter, some of these are discussed with reference to the clinical problems they may cause, either in childhood or later. Following this, renal cystic disease is covered, after which some common acquired paediatric urological conditions are described. The more complex paediatric urological conditions are managed in specialized paediatric surgical units, while many children are managed by a urologist in the setting of a district general hospital.

Common congenital anomalies of the genito-urinary tract

Kidney

Renal anomalies relate to number, position and fusion. Bilateral agenesis, Potter's syndrome is rare and incompatible with life. Unilateral renal agenesis occurs in 1 per 1000 people. The single kidney is usually large and there is no adverse effect on longevity. Supernumerary kidneys are rare.

Renal ectopia

The position of the kidneys, normally on the posterior abdominal wall, may vary according to the site at which their embryological ascent from the pelvis was arrested. Not surprisingly, the commonest site for ectopia is in the pelvis, in 1 in 700 people, usually lying extraperitoneally in the iliac fossa. Rarer ectopias include the thorax and crossing the mid line to fuse onto the normal kidney. Often asymptomatic, problems seen more frequently with ectopic kidneys include hydronephrosis, stones and other GU anomalies.

Horseshoe kidney

The most common fusion anomaly and often asymptomatic, one in 500 people have kidneys that are fused across the midline by an isthmus. This passes in front of the aorta, just below the origin of the inferior mesenteric artery at the level of L4. The ureters pass in front of the isthmus (*Fig. 11.1a*). Other GU anomalies are observed in 30% of individuals. Horseshoes exhibit a characteristic IVU appearance because the renal pelves are rotated forwards. Problems associated with horseshoes include hydronephrosis, stones and renal tumours (*Fig. 11.1b*). Prior to any surgical intervention for these problems, CT scanning and angiography are obtained since the anatomy and blood supply varies from case to case.

Neonatal hydronephrosis

Hydronephrosis is distension of the renal calyces and pelvis with urine, usually due to obstruction at the pelvi-ureteric junction, or distally in the urinary tract. A **pyonephrosis** occurs when the urine has changed to pus in the presence of infection. An incidental finding of hydronephrosis made on routine antenatal ultrasonography presents a dilemma for paediatricians and urologists. In most cases the hydronephrosis settles shortly after birth and should be observed with a renal ultrasound scan within one week of delivery. Those children who have persistent hydronephrosis should be followed with a further ultrasound and dynamic renography. Treatment is discussed below.

Pelvi-ureteric junction (PUJ) obstruction

This is a cause of hydronephrosis, which can be detected at routine antenatal ultrasound, or present clinically during childhood or adult life. The ureter

Fig. 11.1:
(a) Diagram of a normal horseshoe kidney; (b) a contrast-enhanced CT scan showing a horseshoe kidney containing non-enhancing lesions consistent with cysts and tumours.

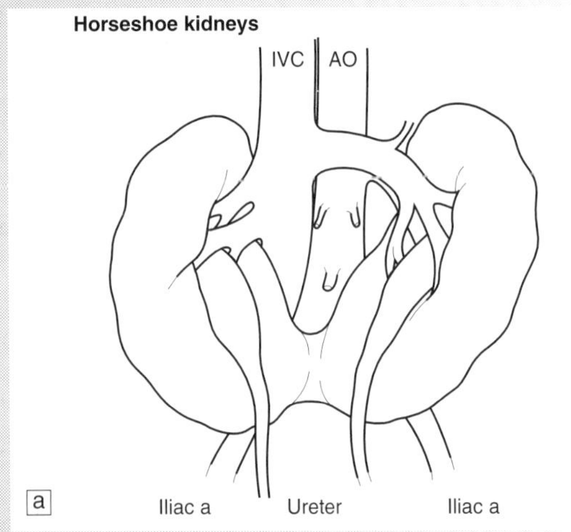

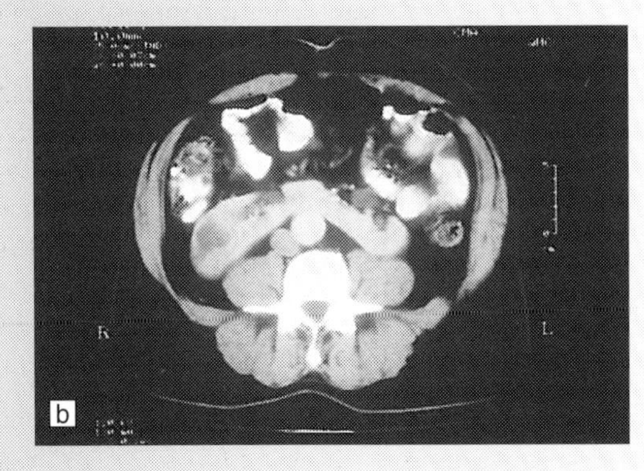

is normal. The PUJ is obstructed either intrinsically by a non-relaxing segment or occasionally a stone, or extrinsically by a lower renal polar artery crossing and compressing it. The clinical presentation in children or young adults, more commonly in males, is with loin pain or urinary tract infections (UTI). If ultrasound demonstrates hydronephrosis, IVU is indicated to assess the ipsilateral ureter and exclude a stone. If no contrast is seen within the ureter, retrograde ureterography is necessary to exclude ureteric obstruction by stone or tumour, particularly in older patients. Finally, before offering surgical treatment, dynamic renography (for example, a MAG3) should be undertaken to prove the hydronephrosis is secondary to obstruction and to document the function of the affected kidney compared to the other (Chapter 2, *Fig. 2.2*). Treatment is surgical: a **pyeloplasty** is performed to incise or excise the obstructing PUJ, reconstructing a widely open new PUJ; an obstructing lower pole vessel is re-routed so that it is no longer compressing. This is accomplished through an extraperitoneal loin incision. Less invasive options include **percutaneous pyelolysis**, which involves making a tract into the renal pelvis and incising the tight PUJ under vision using a nephroscope. The outcomes are inferior to open pyeloplasty. Enthusiasts are developing laparoscopic pyeloplasty: drawbacks to this technique include a steep learning curve for the surgeon and long operating time.

Renal cystic disease

Most renal cysts are congenital and arise from diverticula of obstructed collecting ducts. The collecting ducts may be dilated but not obstructed: this is called **medullary sponge kidney** (MSK). MSK may be focal (confined to a part of one kidney) or diffuse. Patients may develop recurrent UTIs or renal colic due to the formation of tiny calculi in these ducts. The IVU reveals focal or diffuse nephrocalcinosis on the control film and contrast filling the dilated ducts will give a characteristic blush to the affected renal pyramids. There is no specific treatment for MSK.

Adult polycystic kidney disease is an autosomal dominant single-gene (chromosome 16q) disorder, affecting 1 per 1000 births. The kidney shapes are distorted by multiple cysts of varying size, imaged best with ultrasound or CT scans. Cysts occur in other organs; other features include Berry (intracranial) aneurysms and mitral valve prolapse. The disease is often diagnosed on the basis of family history, but is usually not clinically apparent until adulthood. Symptoms include haematuria, loin pain and UTI. Signs include hypertension, renal mass and sometimes hepatomegaly or splenomegaly. Non-imaging investigations reveal anaemia of chronic disease, elevated serum creatinine and proteinuria. Fertility problems occur in patients of both sexes. Management is largely the domain of the nephrologist, aiming to treat hypertension using ACE inhibitors and treat symptoms non-invasively. There are reports of an increased risk of renal neoplasia. By 60 years, half the patients require renal replacement therapy.

Infantile polycystic kidney disease is an autosomal recessive disorder affecting 1 per 10 000 births. The kidneys contain many tiny cysts, so their shape is preserved. Diagnosis is often made on antenatal ultrasound. Hypertension, pulmonary hypoplasia and portal fibrosis are other features. Infants and children develop renal or respiratory failure and many do not survive into adulthood.

Acquired renal cysts

Simple renal cysts occur commonly, with most 60 year-olds having one or more. They may be solitary or multiple. They seldom cause symptoms, or require treatment. Occasionally, a parapelvic cyst might cause PUJ obstruction by extrinsic compression, in which case a trial of ultrasound-guided percutaneous aspiration may be justified, prior to de-roofing the cyst. Renal cysts are seen in patients with **von Hippel Lindau** syndrome (see Chapter 9).

Complex renal cysts are those with radiologically suspicious features. These include calcified or irregular walls and contain solid material. Complex cysts may be malignant and consideration given to nephrectomy (see Chapter 9). Occasionally, infection with the dog tapeworm *Echinococcus granulosus* (**hydatid disease**) gives rise to a renal cyst. These are typically calcified and contain the worms. A history of contact with dogs or sheep would be of help. Serological complement fixation testing is diagnostic. Care should be taken if the cyst requires surgery, because spillage of its contents may cause anaphylaxis. A better treatment is to first inject the cyst with dilute formalin.

Ureteric duplication

Duplication is the most common congenital anomaly of the ureter, observed in 1 in 125 post-mortems, but in 3% of patients undergoing IVU for urinary symptoms. It is bilateral in 40% and more common in females. The renal pelvis may be bifid, draining upper and lower renal poles separately, but join to form a single ureter. Alternatively, two ureters may pass down from the kidney, in which case the ureter draining the upper pole always opens onto the bladder trigone below and medial to the ureter draining the lower pole. A third variant is where the two ureters join at a point along their course to drain into the bladder by a single orifice. While frequently asymptomatic, the clinical problem associated with ureteric duplication is UTI. With incomplete duplication, it is thought that urine can pass from one ureter to the other, rather than draining into the bladder – so-called Yo-Yo reflux. With complete duplications, the ureter draining the lower pole is prone to vesico-ureteric reflux, while the ureter draining the upper pole is prone to development of a ureterocele, which can cause obstruction (*Fig. 11.2b*). Reflux and obstruction both prevent urine from leaving the body, so predispose to infection. Treatment of symptoms refractory to antimicrobials is ureteric re-implantation for reflux and endoscopic incision for ureterocele.

Ectopic ureters are rare. Because of their origin from the mesonephric duct, they can open into the seminal vesicle or epididymis in the male causing recurrent infections at those sites in boys, or into the vagina, distal to the urinary sphincter, causing incontinence in girls.

Ureterocele

A ureterocele is a cystic dilatation of the distal ureter as it drains into the bladder, seen in 1 per 4000 people (*Fig. 11.2a*). They can be found in single systems (orthotopic), or more often associated with the upper pole ureter of a duplex system (ectopic – *Fig. 11.2b*). Both are four times more common in females. Children and adults may present with UTI, or ureteroceles may be observed incidentally on ultrasound scanning. Rarely, examination of the female introitus can reveal a prolapsing ureterocele coming through the urethra, presenting as an interlabial mass. Further investigation should include an IVU or renography to assess the renal function prior to offering treatment. If the renal function is satisfactory, treatment is by

Fig. 11.2:
(a) An ultrasound scan showing a dilated distal ureter passing behind the bladder associated with a ureterocele; (b) a diagram showing a duplex ureter with an upper pole ectopic ureterocele.

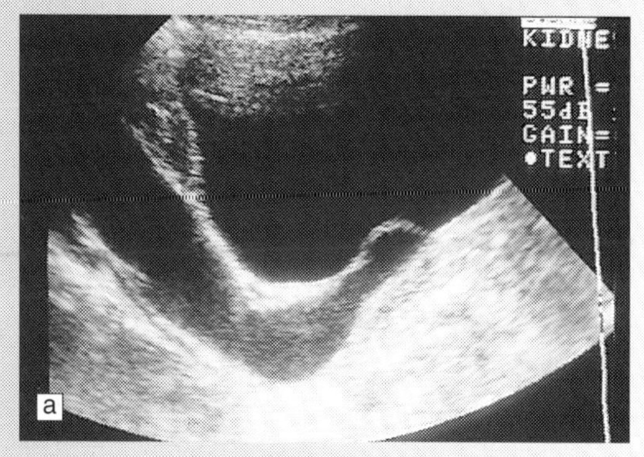

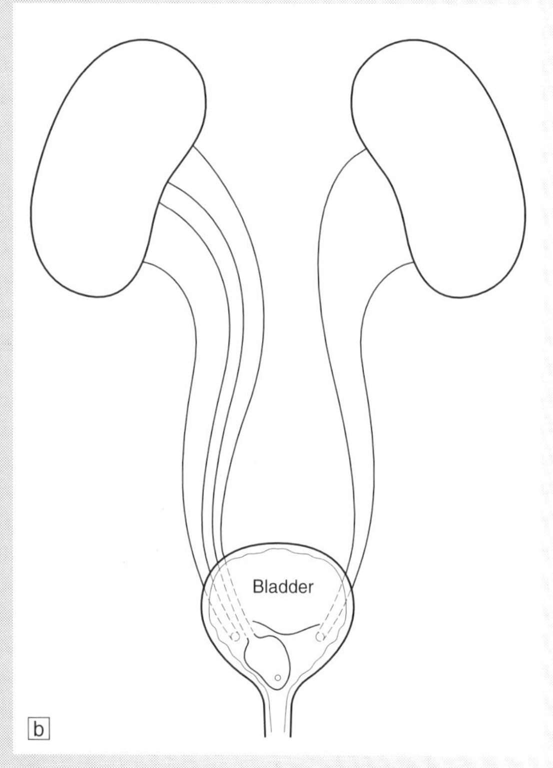

endoscopic transurethral incision, allowing drainage. Alternatively, for chronic poorly functioning pyelonephritic upper renal poles, partial nephroureterectomy is indicated.

Vesico-ureteric reflux

Vesico-ureteric reflux (VUR) refers to regurgitation of urine from the bladder up the ureter, sometimes to the kidney. It may be primary, or secondary to a neurogenic bladder. Primary VUR occurs in up to 1% of children, five times more commonly in girls and there is often a family history. The cause is a poorly supported distal ureter and as such is commonly associated with lower pole duplex ureters. The commonest presentation is a child with a UTI. **50% of children with UTI have reflux, hence any child with pyelonephritis, any boy or any girl <5 years with UTI and any girl >5 years with two or more episodes of cystitis require investigation with an MCUG and renal ultrasound**. At cystoscopy, refluxing ureteric orifices look like golf holes. Reflux can cause renal scarring secondary to infection, which may result in hypertension or end-stage renal failure if not treated. Scarring is best assessed by static renography. However, most patients with VUR can be managed conservatively with regular timed voiding and antimicrobial prophylaxis, since spontaneous resolution of the VUR commonly occurs later in childhood. Ureteric re-implantation (or endoscopic subtrigonal injection of the ureteric orifice) is indicated for children with severe reflux, breakthrough UTIs, evidence of progressive renal scarring and VUR that persists into teenage life. If the VUR is secondary to a high-pressure neurogenic bladder, this must be treated prior to anti-reflux surgery.

Bladder exstrophy

Previously termed ectopia vesicae, this dreadful malformation is characterized by the bladder exposed onto the lower anterior abdominal wall and epispadias (*Fig. 11.3*), associated with inguinal herniae, a widened pubic symphysis and VUR. It appears to be caused by failure of medial mesenchymal migration to form the abdominal wall and tubularize the embryonic bladder. It occurs in 1 in 50 000 births, more commonly in boys. **Epispadias** is a penile malformation characterized by the urethral meatus opening proximally and on the dorsal surface, instead of ventrally (*Fig. 11.4*).

Fig. 11.3:
A rare example of untreated bladder exstrophy and epispadias in an adult.

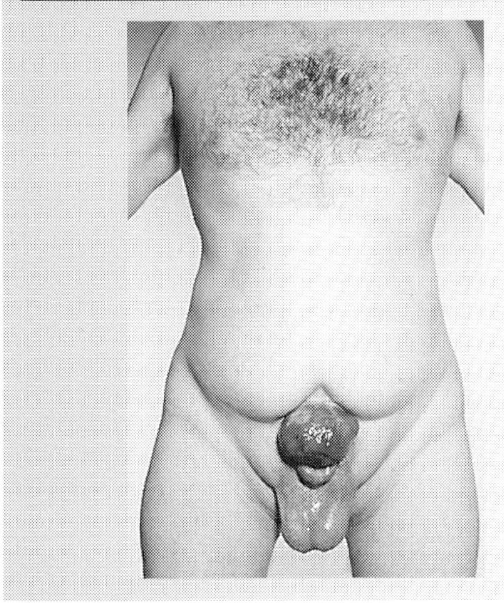

Fig. 11.4:
An epispadias in a child whose bladder exstrophy has previously been closed. The flat urethral plate was tubularized and distally brought through the penile corpora cavernosa so the meatus finished in a ventral position on the glans.

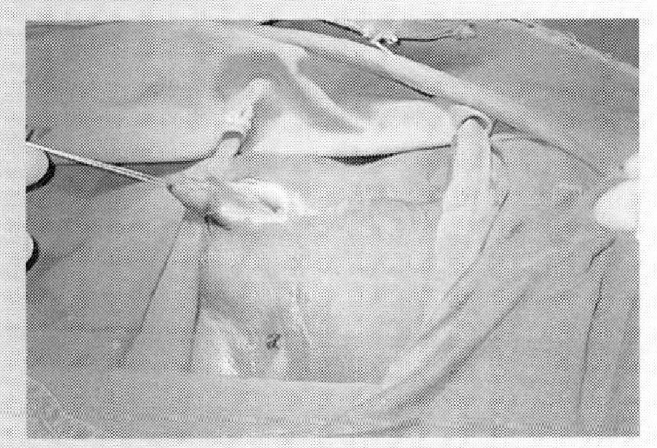

Female epispadias is characterized by a bifid clitoris and duplex vagina. The diagnosis is obvious on examination of the infant's abdomen. The bladder should be covered with a sterile wrap and the infant referred to a specialist centre. Here, the bladder is closed, the bladder neck reconstructed and the epispadias repaired. Late complications include incontinence, uterine prolapse during pregnancy and adenocarcinoma (see Chapter 9). A more severe variant is **cloacal exstrophy**, where there is also exposed detubularized gut on the abdominal wall.

Prune belly syndrome

This syndrome is seen in 1 in 50 000 births, characterized by abnormal development of the anterior abdominal wall, which looks wrinkled like the skin of a prune (*Fig. 11.5*). There are numerous associated GU, pulmonary, cardiac, gastrointestinal and musculoskeletal abnormalities, since it is due to some abnormality in the differentiation of embryonic mesenchyme. Undescended testes, hypoplastic kidneys, megaureters, urachal fistula and dilated prostatic urethra are described associations. A total of 25% of patients develop renal failure.

Posterior urethral valves

Posterior urethral valves (PUV) occur in 1 per 8000 male births. They are mucosal folds in the prostatic

Fig. 11.5:
A baby with prune belly syndrome, and a catheter inserted through a patent urachal fistula.

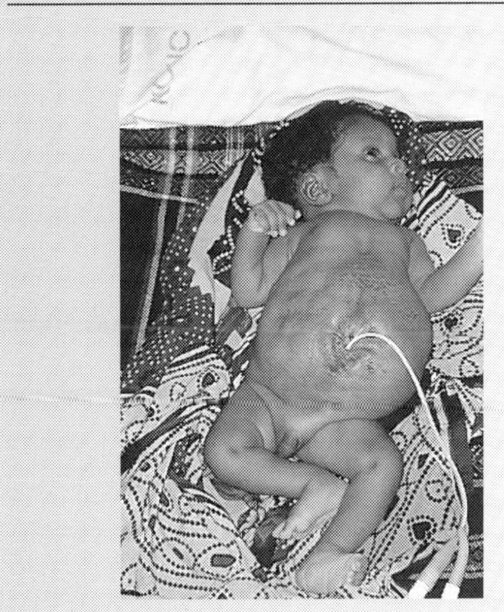

urethra that cause BOO in the fetus and beyond (*Fig. 11.6*). Antenatal ultrasound performed for oligohydramnios will demonstrate bilateral hydronephrosis and a thick-walled full bladder. If not detected then, infant boys develop UTI, urinary ascites or respiratory distress due to the associated pulmonary hypoplasia. Clinically, the bladder is palpated suprapubically where it feels like a walnut. Older boys, with lesser degrees of BOO, present with daytime incontinence. At diagnosis, the renal function is assessed by renography and serum creatinine and electrolytes. Acidosis and hyperkalaemia are common. The renal function is stabilized by insertion of a fine catheter and subsequently the PUVs are incised endoscopically. Unfortunately, this is not often the end of the problem and close follow-up is required. A neurogenic bladder is still present, so VUR is often demonstrated by a MCUG. End-stage pulmonary disease or renal failure are common sequelae.

Undescended testis (UDT)

Present in approximately 4% of full-term neonates and 1% of boys at one year, the exact cause of UDT is not clear but it may be related to abnormal development of the gubernaculum and epididymis and fetal androgen levels. One third are bilateral.

Fig. 11.6:
A cystogram of a male infant showing a dilated prostatic urethra typically seen in the presence of posterior urethral valves.

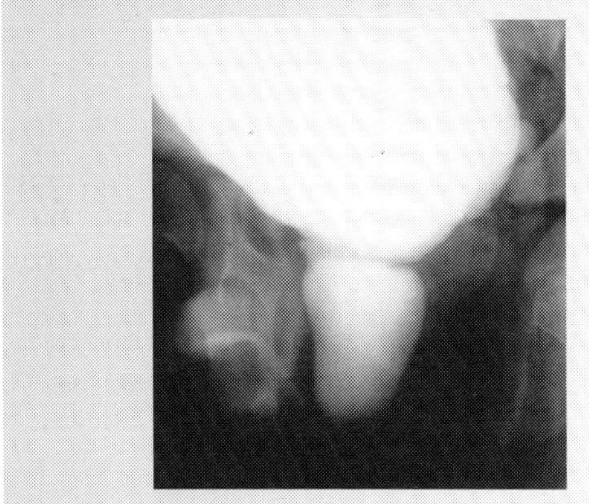

UDT may be arrested along the line of descent from the posterior abdominal wall (cryptorchidism) or located in an abnormal site (ectopic), such as the perineum (*Fig. 11.7*). 65% of cryptorchid testes are located in the inguinal canal, of which 80% are palpable.

Clinical examination should distinguish a retractile testis from a UDT. A retractile testis is one that can easily be brought down into a scrotal position when the child is relaxed (ideally squatting) or under anaesthetic; treatment is not required. The UDT will require orchidopexy, which is fixation in

Fig. 11.7:
The undescended testis. (a) Ectopic sites; (b) cryptorchid sites.

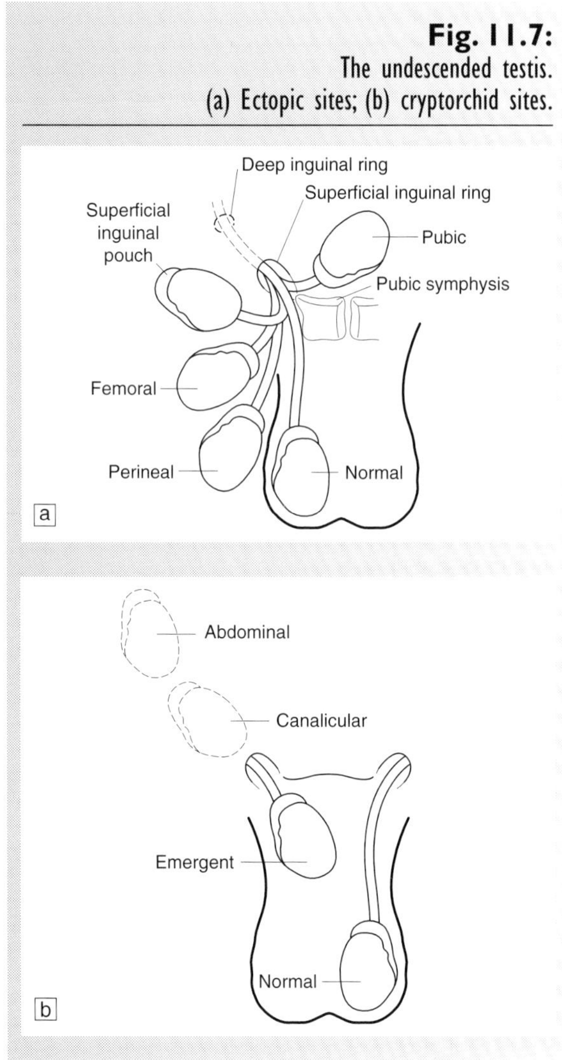

the scrotum with two or three non-absorbable sutures. If examination fails to reveal a palpable testis, an ultrasound of the groin, an MRI scan of the posterior abdominal wall, or a laparoscopy is indicated to locate the testis.

It is current practice to perform orchidopexy by the age of 2 years. This goes some way to preventing long-term complications of UDT, which include **infertility**, testicular **torsion** and a 10-fold increased risk of **testicular cancer** later in life. There is also a smaller increased risk of the normally descended contralateral testis developing cancer. 50% of torted UDT are associated with cancer. If an adult of >30 years presents with UDT, consideration should be given to offering orchidectomy or imaging surveillance, wherever the site.

Hypospadias

This is the commonest congenital penile anomaly, affecting 1 in 400 male infants. The urethral meatus opens at some site on the ventral surface of the penis between the penoscrotal junction and the normal site at the tip of the glans, reflecting underdevelopment of the urethral plate. The meatus is most commonly (70%) sited at the glans or coronal sulcus (*Fig. 11.8*). There is usually an associated hooded foreskin and chordee (ventral penile curvature), but surprisingly there is no association with other GU anomalies. However, severe hypospadias in the presence of cryptorchidism should raise the possibility of congenital adrenal hyperplasia (CAH, below). Surgical reconstruction of the urethra is recommended at 12–24 months of age, to avoid cosmetic and fertility problems in adulthood. Urethrocutaneous fistula complicates 10% of these procedures.

Fig. 11.8: Glanular hypospadias, ventral and lateral views, illustrating the position of the meatus, the hooded foreskin and the ventral chordee.

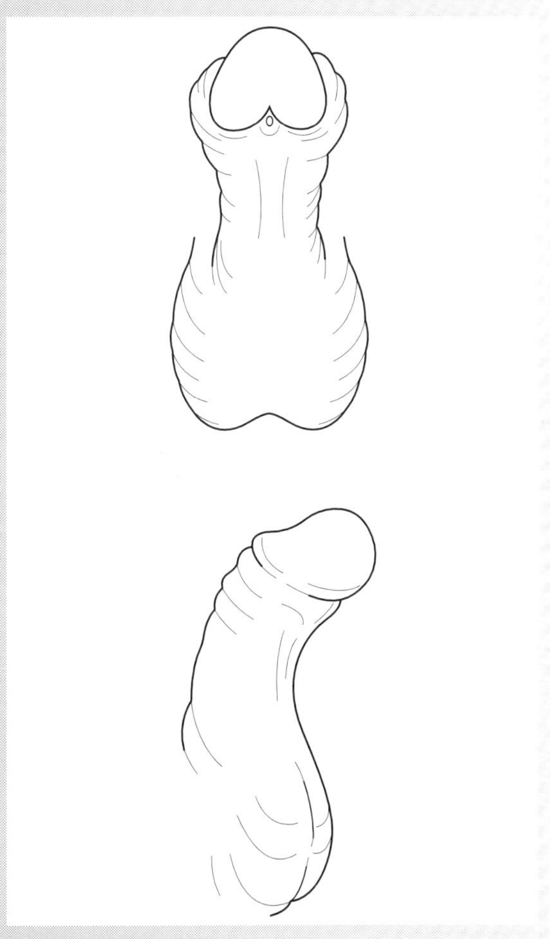

Redrawn from *Essential Urology 1st Edn.*, Bullock *et al.*, Fig. 6.6, 1989, by permission of the publisher Churchill Livingstone.

Ambiguous genitalia

One per 10 000 births has ambiguous genitalia, causing difficulties assigning the sex. The genitalia of all male newborns should be assessed for the presence of palpable gonads (always testes), phallus size and the location of the urethra. The finding of AG should prompt investigation by karyotyping, a serum 17-hydroxyprogesterone level, pelvic ultrasound, laparoscopy and gonadal biopsy. This is a complex and specialized area within paediatric urology.

A true hermaphrodite has both ovarian and testicular tissue. The karyotype is either 46XX or 46XY with mosaicism. The child is usually brought up as a male.

The commonest cause of female pseudohermaphroditism is congenital adrenal hyperplasia (CAH). Here, due to an inborn enzyme deficiency relating to steroid metabolism, the adrenals are secreting vast quantities of androgen, virilizing the female fetus. Clinical features are cryptorchidism and penoscrotal hypospadias due to clitoral masculinization. An elevated serum concentration of 17-hydroxyprogesterone is diagnostic. The most serious problem with CAH is the salt-wasting nephropathy due to absent production of aldosterone and cortisol, requiring life-saving hormone replacement. Reconstructive surgery is required later to the clitoris and vagina. Maternal progestagen ingestion during pregnancy may result in female pseudohermaphroditism.

The commonest cause of male pseudohermaphroditism is testicular feminization syndrome. Here, a male fetus has a female phenotype due to androgen insensitivity, often with palpable testes. Often unsuspected until the teenager is undergoing investigation for amenorrhoea, the serum LH and testosterone are elevated.

Acquired conditions

Phimosis

At birth, **preputial adhesions** are often present between the glans penis and foreskin but under normal circumstances separation occurs by the age of 10 years. Most prepuces are fully retractile by 2 years of age but some adolescents may retain some minor adhesions. Scarring of the foreskin may develop causing inability to retract it. This is called **phimosis**, most frequently due to balanitis xerotica obliterans (BXO), a fibrosing condition of unknown aetiology, which can also cause stenosis of the urethral meatus.

Phimosis may cause recurrent infection beneath the foreskin (balanitis) or a significant reduction in the urinary stream with ballooning of the foreskin. Phimosis may also hide a squamous carcinoma in older men who neglect their genitalia. The treatment of phimosis is **circumcision**, though some surgeons perform the unsightly dorsal slit procedure. Circumcision is one of the oldest operations in history, described by the ancient Egyptians. Only 2% of young adult men have a phimosis, yet historically 6% have had a circumcision by this age, so it appears we were doing too many. There is still a tendency to be asked by parents or young men for circumcision when there is no evidence of a phimosis. General anaesthesia is commonly given, though circumcision may be performed under local anaesthetic if necessary. Complications include a 2% chance of haematoma and a 'buried penis' if too much skin is inadvertently removed. The foreskin should be submitted for histology, since the finding of BXO justifies a warning to the patient about possible future development of meatal stenosis. Circumcision is performed on religious grounds for Muslim boys, Jews, Ethiopian Christians and other groups, usually not by urologists.

Paraphimosis

A urological emergency, this is the painful result of retraction of a phimosis. If the foreskin is not reduced in a timely fashion, it constricts the glans, causing pain and swelling (*Fig. 11.9*). The longer this continues, the more difficult it is to reduce. The two commonest scenarios are of a man who has had intercourse, falls asleep and wakes with the problem; or of a patient whose foreskin was retracted to be cleaned prior to catheterization, but not reduced afterwards. Treatment is first by administering analgesia and local anaesthetic, then squeezing the glans for 2–3 minutes to reduce the swelling, before attempting to reduce the oedematous foreskin. A technique of making tiny punctures in the oedematous foreskin using a fine

Fig. 11.9:
Paraphimosis. This patient is about to undergo an emergency circumcision.

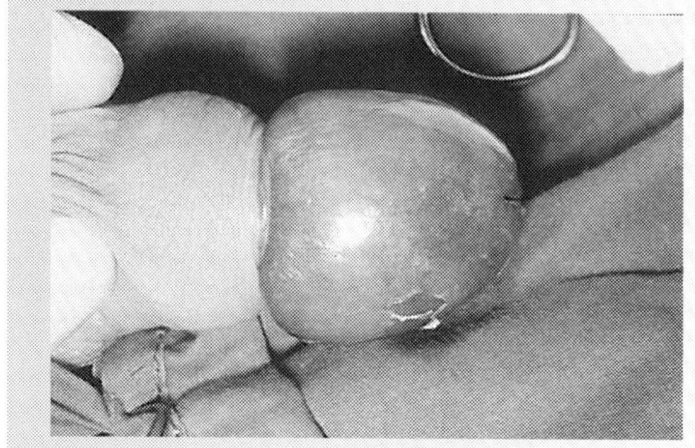

needle prior to reduction has been described. If all else fails, an emergency circumcision is required.

Childhood UTI

Asymptomatic bacteriuria is observed in 2.5% of children <2 years old and 1% of schoolchildren. The significance of this is unclear. One percent of boys and 5% of girls develop a UTI during school years. There are several risk factors for UTI, including VUR (see page 128), female sex, constipation and the foreskin.

Symptoms of cystitis or pyelonephritis are often easy to elicit and investigate by sending an MSU for culture. However, if the patient is an infant, the symptoms are less specific: fever, irritability, poor feeding, vomiting and diarrhoea. So the diagnosis of UTI should be considered in any child with a fever and vomiting ... then there is the difficulty of obtaining a clean urine sample for stick-testing as well as considering all the other possible causes of the symptoms.

Treatment for UTI not associated with reflux is with antimicrobials: 5 days for cystitis and 14 days for pyelonephritis. A well-absorbed broad-spectrum agent such as amoxycillin (syrup or capsules) is ideal unless vomiting precludes oral administration, in which case a combination of intravenous gentamicin and ampicillin is excellent. These should be continued prophylactically if recurrent UTI occurs despite normal radiological investigation. This may help prevent renal scarring and the development of chronic pyelonephritis.

Stones

Renal calculi are rare in childhood. They may present with loin pain, UTI or haematuria. Investigations will include an ultrasound and plain KUB radiograph, or an IVU. Treatment is the same as for adults – see Chapter 8.

Tumours

Tumours of the GU tract in children are rare but those most commonly seen include Wilms' tumour of the kidney and rhabdomyosarcomas of the prostate, bladder and paratesticular tissue. Children presenting with an abdominal mass, with or without haematuria, should be investigated with an abdominal CT scan. The management of Wilms' tumour is discussed in Chapter 9. Radical surgery is usually indicated for non-metastatic rhabdomyosarcoma, combined with chemotherapy and radiotherapy.

Key points

- PUJ obstruction can occur in all age-groups and is a common cause of hydronephrosis. It is usually due to a congenital failure of relaxation of the PUJ muscle, but extrinsic compression by a renal artery or intrinsic obstruction by a stone or tumour are possibilities.
- With complete duplications, the ureter draining the lower pole is prone to vesico-ureteric reflux, while the ureter draining the upper pole is prone to development of a utereocele, which can cause obstruction.
- Any boy or girl <5 years with UTI and any girl >5 years with two or more episodes of cystitis require investigation with an MCUG and renal ultrasound, since 50% will have vesico-ureteric reflux.
- Only 2% of young adult men have a phimosis, yet historically 6% have had a circumcision by this age.
- The foreskin should always be reduced following examination or urethral catheterization to prevent development of a paraphimosis.
- Long-term complications of undescended testis include infertility, testicular torsion and a 10-fold increased risk of testicular cancer (seminoma) in later life.

Cases

1. A 4-year-old girl complains of pain in the right flank and burning when she passes urine. She has vomited once. Her temperature is 38°C and her abdomen is soft, though she is tender in the right renal angle.
   (a) What is the likely diagnosis?
   (b) Which investigations and treatment are required immediately?
   (c) What further management is indicated?

2. A 15-year-old youth complains of bouts of left loin pain, lasting 2–3 hours, every few days. These started three months previously, after a family wedding when he evidently consumed a large quantity of lemonade. He is missing some school lessons because of the pain. He has no LUTS. Examination is unremarkable.
   (a) What is the likely diagnosis?
   (b) Which investigations are indicated?
   (c) What if the investigations are normal?

Answers

1. (a) This little girl probably has a UTI complicated with right pyelonephritis. The differential diagnosis should include appendicitis, but her abdomen shows no rigidity, guarding or rebound tenderness.
   (b) A clean catch urine, ideally MSU, is collected, stick-tested and sent for microscopy, culture and sensitivity. Paracetamol is given to reduce the pyrexia. Amoxycillin syrup is prescribed for 14 days and she is reviewed the following day. Fortunately, there has been an improvement in the pain, with no further vomiting. The MSU grew 10^5 colonies ml^{-1} of *E. coli*, sensitive to amoxycillin.
   (c) Referral is made to a paediatrician, who arranges an urgent outpatient appointment. He is interested in the family history, considering the possibility of VUR. The girl's blood pressure is checked and is normal. A renal ultrasound and a MCUG are arranged. The ultrasound is normal, but the MCUG shows slight VUR into the right ureter. This is managed conservatively, but six months later she develops another UTI. This time, the antimicrobials are continued at a low-dose prophylactically. A DMSA renogram shows no signs of renal scarring. The little girl's prognosis is good, with every chance that her VUR will resolve over the next few years.

2. (a) The diagnosis in a boy this age is intermittent PUJ obstruction. The differential diagnosis should include renal colic due to stone and musculoskeletal pain.
   (b) He should have a renal ultrasound, IVU and a dynamic MAG3 renogram. The diagnosis is suggested if the ultrasound demonstrates a left hydronephrosis, confirmed with IVU and renography.
   (c) If these investigations are normal, a repeat MAG3 renogram with administration of frusemide 15 minutes prior to injection of the isotope. This causes a diuresis which may precipitate the problem, just like the lemonade did! Even better, the renogram could be repeated during an attack of pain. He had the former option, which demonstrated obstruction on the left. A pyeloplasty was performed through a flank incision, at which a lower pole artery was kinking the PUJ. The PUJ was dismembered, the tight area excised and the PUJ reconstructed over a ureteric stent, placing the artery the other side of the PUJ, no longer compressing it. The stent was removed transurethrally 6 weeks later and no more pain after lemonade has been reported.

Further Reading

Gillenwater J., Grayhack J.T., Howards S.S. and Duckett J.W. (1996). *Adult and Paediatric Urology*. Third edition. Mosby, St Louis.

Moore K.L. and Persaud T.V. (1998). *The Developing Human: Clinically-Orientated Embryology*. Sixth edition. Saunders, London.

Resnick M.D. and Novick, A.C. (1995). *Urology Secrets*. Hanley & Belfus, Philadelphia.

CHAPTER 12

Renal failure and renal transplantation

Introduction

Renal failure can be treated by dialysis or transplantation. Transplantation is now a common procedure and generally accepted as the best form of treatment for end stage renal failure (ESRF). Joseph Murray and his colleagues carried out the first successful human kidney allograft between identical twins in Boston in 1954. It was met with spectacular success because it bypassed the immunological problems of rejection since it took place between one identical twin and another. For his pioneering work in transplantation, Joseph Murray shared the Nobel Prize for Medicine in 1990. Apart from results with identical twins the early days of transplantation were fraught with poor results due to the problems of rejection. While this is still a major problem, a number of factors, including the advent of modern immunosuppressive drugs have improved the results considerably. A passage is included in this chapter on retroperitoneal fibrosis.

Renal failure

Renal failure may be acute or chronic. Acute renal failure may be pre-renal, renal or post renal and the common causes are outlined in *Table 12.1*.

Pre-renal and renal causes have a prodromal phase where some urine is formed. It is often cloudy and contains debris and casts. After the prodromal phase urine may or may not be produced. If it is, it is dilute and in both situations, creatinine and urea are not cleared and build up in the blood, along with potassium. Complete obstruction leads to anuria. During the recovery phase, and/or after relief of obstruction, a large diuresis takes place, and during this time it is important to keep the patient hydrated, which will often require intravenous fluids with replacement of electrolytes, especially sodium. Temporary dialysis may be necessary until the kidneys recover.

Chronic renal failure (CRF) is the permanent loss of renal function, which eventually may lead to end stage renal failure. ESRF affects between 60–160 people per million of the population. Acute renal failure, which does not recover, will progress to chronic renal failure, and other causes of ESRF are shown in *Table 12.2*.

The rate of deterioration in chronic renal failure may be slow, and in this situation diet alone has an important role to play in limiting the protein intake which in turn limits the build up of urea in the blood. Chronic renal failure leads to a series of clinical features as outlined in *Table 12.3*.

Table 12.1:
Causes of acute renal failure

Type	Cause	Example
Pre-renal	Poor renal perfusion	Blood loss, sepsis, drugs (e.g. angiotensin-converting enzyme [ACE] inhibitors, and non-steroidal anti-inflammatory agents)
Renal	Tubular damage	Crush injury (myoglobin), mismatched transfusion (haemoglobin), poison (mercury, clostridium toxin)
Post-renal	Obstruction	Bilateral ureteric obstruction (stone, tumour, retroperitoneal fibrosis or surgical injury); unilateral obstruction in a solitary kidney.

Table 12.2:
The aetiology of ESRF

Cause	Percentage
Chronic glomerulonephritis	25
Chronic pyelonephritis	15
Diabetes	12
Unknown	13
Miscellaneous (including retroperitoneal fibrosis)	12
Hypertension	10
Polycystic disease	8
Analgesic nephropathy	5

Investigations of renal failure

The urine is examined for haematuria, proteinuria and looked at microscopically for casts. The amount of proteinuria is assessed over a 24-hour peroid. Red blood cells can be examined microscopically. Fragmented or dysmorphic red cells point to a glomerular origin and are seen in such diseases as proliferative glomerulonephritis and immunoglobulin A nephropathy. Ultrasound scan looks at the size of the kidneys and will identify hydronephrosis. A plain abdominal X-ray may show stones in the line of the urinary tract. Computerized tomography can look in more detail at stone disease and the presence of obstruction. An angiogram, CT or MRI angiogram will identify renovascular disease. A renal biopsy may be indicated.

Dialysis and access surgery

In the days before dialysis and transplantation, end stage renal failure led to death. Dialysis was developed in the 1930s and today is carried out in one of two ways.

Chronic ambulatory peritoneal dialysis (CAPD) is carried out by means of a silicon (Tenckhoff) catheter inserted into the abdominal cavity. The dialysate fluid runs through multiple side holes into the abdomen, left for several hours and then is allowed to drain out. It can be carried out in many places (*Fig. 12.1*).

CAPD is not possible if there has been a lot of previous abdominal surgery with adhesions. The major complication of CAPD is peritonitis, the risk being one episode per year per patient. *Staphylococcus* is the usual organism, but Gram-negative sepsis may occur from the bowel, especially in patients with diverticular disease. Hernias can occur at the port of entry and occasionally genital oedema is seen, sometimes due to a peritoneal leak.

Haemodialysis takes blood from the patient which is allowed to flow over a dialysing membrane. This allows the solutes to pass into the dialysis fluid so purifying the blood. Today the common method is to create a peripheral fistula whereby an artery and vein (usually radial artery and cephalic

Table 12.3:
Clinical features of chronic renal failure

Clinical feature	Cause
Anaemia	Loss of erythropoietin as renal tissue is destroyed
Neuropathy	Loss of myelin from peripheral nerves
Pericarditis	High urea levels
Osteomalacia	Decreased calcium absorption from gut due to vitamin D insensitivity
Secondary hyperparathyroidism	Phosphate accumulates, calcium falls, parathyroid hormone-stimulated ectopic calcification

Fig. 12.1:
CAPD can be carried out in many situations.

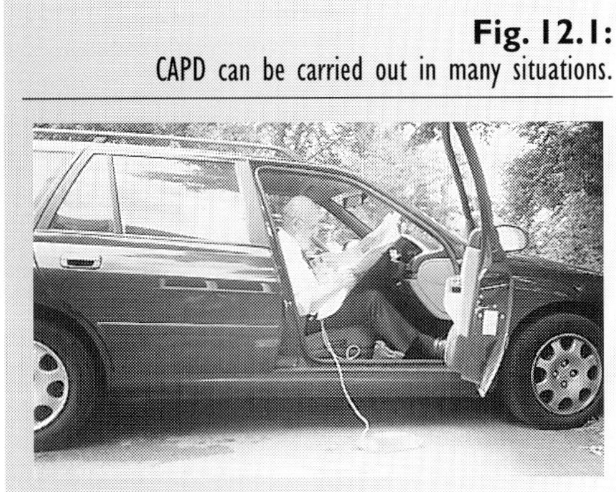

vein) are anastomosed (*Fig. 12.2*). This creates a large hypertrophied vessel that can be repeatedly needled allowing blood to be diverted into a dialysis machine, purified and recirculated back to the patient. Although the current forms of haemodialysis are much more efficient than the early days, complications still occur. These can be due to the underlying problems associated with ESRF and the specific complications of dialysis. Death from myocardial infarction is 20 times higher in dialysis patients due to hyperlipidaemia, hypertension and left ventricular hypertrophy. Renal osteodystrophy, amyloidosis and anaemia are common. Malignancy, hepatitis and tuberculosis are more common due to the immuno-compromised nature of patients in ESRF. Other infections can enter via the dialysis catheters. Fistulas may thrombose due to dehydration and decreased blood flow.

Fig. 12.2:
Radio-cephalic fistula.

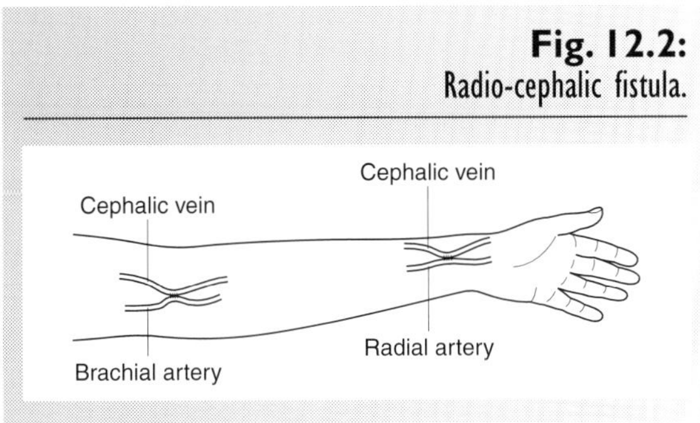

Retroperitoneal fibrosis

Introduction

Retroperitoneal fibrosis was first clearly described by the French urologist, Albarran, at the beginning of the twentieth century as 'stenosing periureteritis'. In 1948 Ormond described two patients with diffuse fibrosis of the retroperitoneal tissues who presented with backache, anaemia and anuria, and he established the clinical and pathological entity of idiopathic retroperitoneal fibrosis. An increasing number of causes of retroperitoneal fibrosis are now recognized and can be divided into benign and malignant.

Benign

Idiopathic retroperitoneal fibrosis comprises two thirds of the benign cases. A fibrous plaque extends laterally and downwards from the renal arteries encasing the aorta, inferior vena cava and ureters, but rarely extends into the pelvis. The central portion of the plaque consists of woody scar tissue, while the growing margins have the histological appearance of chronic inflammation. Although no aetiological factor is usually identified, drugs implicated include methysergide, which was taken for migraine, betablockers, haloperidol, amphetamines and LSD. Occasionally, chronic urinary infections including TB, or inflammatory conditions such as Crohn's disease or sarcoidosis, can lead to retroperitoneal fibrosis. There is an association between abdominal aortic aneurysm (AAA) and idiopathic fibrosis: this may be due to periaortitis, haemorrhage or an immune response to insoluble lipoprotein. More recently it has been described as a complication of intra-arterial stents and angioplasty.

Malignant

Lymphoma is the most common malignant tumour presenting as retroperitoneal fibrosis. **Carcinomas** of the breast, stomach, pancreas, colon, bladder, prostate and carcinoid tumours may be associated with retroperitoneal fibrosis due to metastasis or local infiltration. **Radiotherapy** for the treatment of cancer may cause retroperitoneal fibrosis, although this is much less common today with more precise field localization.

Chemotherapy, especially following treatment of metastatic testicular tumours, may leave fibrous retroperitoneal masses encasing the ureters. These may or may not contain residual tumour, and may require surgical excision.

Presentation

Idiopathic retroperitoneal fibrosis classically affects males in the fifth or sixth decade of life. Men are affected twice as commonly as women. In the early stage, presentation is relatively non-specific, including loss of appetite and weight, fever, sweating and malaise. Dull, non-colicky abdominal pain is described in up to 90% of patients. Later, the major complication of the disease develops: bilateral ureteric obstruction, causing anuria and renal failure. Examination may reveal hypertension in up to 60% of patients and an underlying cause such as an abdominal aortic aneurysm.

Investigations

Classically the erythrocyte sedimentation rate (ESR) is elevated. Pyuria or bacteriuria are commonly found. Ultrasound will demonstrate uni- or bilateral hydronephrosis and proximal hydroureter. Typical features on IVU or ureterography are medial displacement of the ureters with proximal dilatation. Up to one third of patients will have a non-functioning kidney at the time of presentation due to longstanding obstruction. Both CT scanning and MRI can define the area of fibrosis precisely. Fine needle biopsy of the mass may be helpful in confirming the presence of malignant disease, but a negative result does not exclude malignancy.

Management

The **emergency management** of a patient presenting with established renal failure requires relief of the obstruction by percutaneous nephrostomy or ureteric stenting. Monitoring and replacement of fluid and electrolyte losses following relief of bilateral ureteric obstruction is vital: daily weighing and measurement of blood pressure lying and standing are good practice. The underlying cause is investigated as described above. **Spontaneous resolution** of retroperitoneal fibrosis without treatment is a rare occurrence. **Steroids** may decrease the oedema often associated with retroperitoneal fibrosis and in this way help reduce the obstruction. If used, they are usually discontinued when the ESR returns to normal. More recently, the anti-oestrogen **tamoxifen** has been used successfully in some patients, and cyclophosphamide has been reported to have some benefit. **Surgical treatment** (ureterolysis) is often necessary to free the ureters from the encasing fibrous tissue. At the time, biopsies are taken to exclude malignancy. After freeing the ureters from the fibrous sheath surrounding them, the omentum is wrapped around the ureters throughout their length, keeping them free of fibrous tissue. Follow-up with serum creatinine and ultrasound is important to monitor for recurrent disease, although bilateral ureterolysis usually has a satisfactory outcome.

Renal transplantation

Terminology

The term 'transplantation' like its synonym 'graft' was borrowed by surgeons from horticulture. *Table 12.4* describes the different terms used in transplantation.

Problems of supply and demand

With an increasing number of patients on dialysis, and a relaxation in the criteria for accepting patients on to a transplant waiting list, the shortage of available organs is one of the major problems facing transplant surgeons today. While the number of cadaveric kidney transplants in the UK increased from 814 in 1981 to 1736 in 1990, even that failed to prevent the waiting list for those requiring a transplant growing from around 2000 to just under 4000 in the same period of time. The current waiting list is now over 6000 (partly as a result of first and second grafts failing over time) while the transplant rate has remained steady at 1700 cadaveric transplants per year. This is in part due to the drop in fatal road traffic accidents, which is of course very good news on this front. A number of solutions to this problem have been discussed but one area that has increased over the last few years is increasing the number of living related and unrelated (mainly husband/wife) donors.

Table 12.4:
Terminology of transplantation

Terminology	Definition	Example
Autotransplantation	An organ is transplanted into a different site in the same individual	A kidney with a long section of damaged ureter moved down to the iliac fossa
Allotransplantation	Transplantation of an organ from one individual to another of the same species	Any organ transplant from one person to another – most current organ transplants
Xenotransplantation	Transplantation between different species	Organ transplants from animals to humans
Heterotopic	Transplant away from native site	All kidney transplants – into iliac fossa usually leaving native kidneys in place
Orthotopic	Transplant into normal anatomic site after removal of diseased organ	All liver transplants

Donor surgery

Kidneys may be retrieved from living or cadaveric donors. Living donors are usually related but may be unrelated, such as husband to wife. Cadaveric donors are usually on a ventilator and have been diagnosed as brain dead after suffering from an intra-cerebral catastrophe. The role of the transplant coordinator in this situation is crucial and the flow chart (*Fig. 12.3*) shows how the donor is managed.

Renal perfusion solution

In the case of living related donors, the kidney is perfused immediately after removal from the donor. In the case of cadaveric donors, other organs are usually removed as well, and the organs are perfused in situ by a specially designed perfusion solution at 4°C. This marks the start of cold ischaemic time. The purpose of perfusion at this temperature is to decrease the kidney's metabolic and oxygen demands by 95% as well as flushing the donor's blood out of the kidney. There are several solutions that can be used for kidney perfusion and preservation. These have evolved over the last 30 years and vary in solute composition, but all are solutions of similar consistency to intra-cellular fluid, rich in potassium adenosine sugar and ATP. One of the most common is University of Wisconsin (UW) solution, which is suitable for simultaneous perfusion of the kidney, liver and pancreas in the case of multi-organ donors.

Cadaveric donor surgery

Most cadaveric donors today are multi-organ donors and consent is given for removal of heart, lungs, liver and kidneys. A careful laparotomy is carried out to exclude occult neoplasm. After in situ perfusion of the organs, the kidneys can be removed either en bloc or separately. A patch of aortic wall (Carrel patch) is excised with the renal artery to facilitate the arterial anastomosis onto the recipient's external iliac artery. The right renal vein is harvested together with a segment of the inferior vena cava for lengthening the right renal vein if necessary. Particular attention is given to the careful removal of the ureters, with preservation of the peri-ureteric tissue to prevent ischaemia to the lower end of the ureter which after transplantation is dependent solely on the blood supply from the renal artery. The kidneys are then packed in slush and stored at 4°C. This period of time is known as the cold ischaemic time, and in the ideal situation the kidneys are transplanted in less than 24 hours.

The upper age limit for cadaveric donors has been rising over the years and now 20% are over the age of 60. Congenital abnormalities in renal donors are not necessarily a contra-indication to transplantation. Duplex kidneys and horseshoe

Fig. 12.3:
Management of the cadaveric kidney donor.

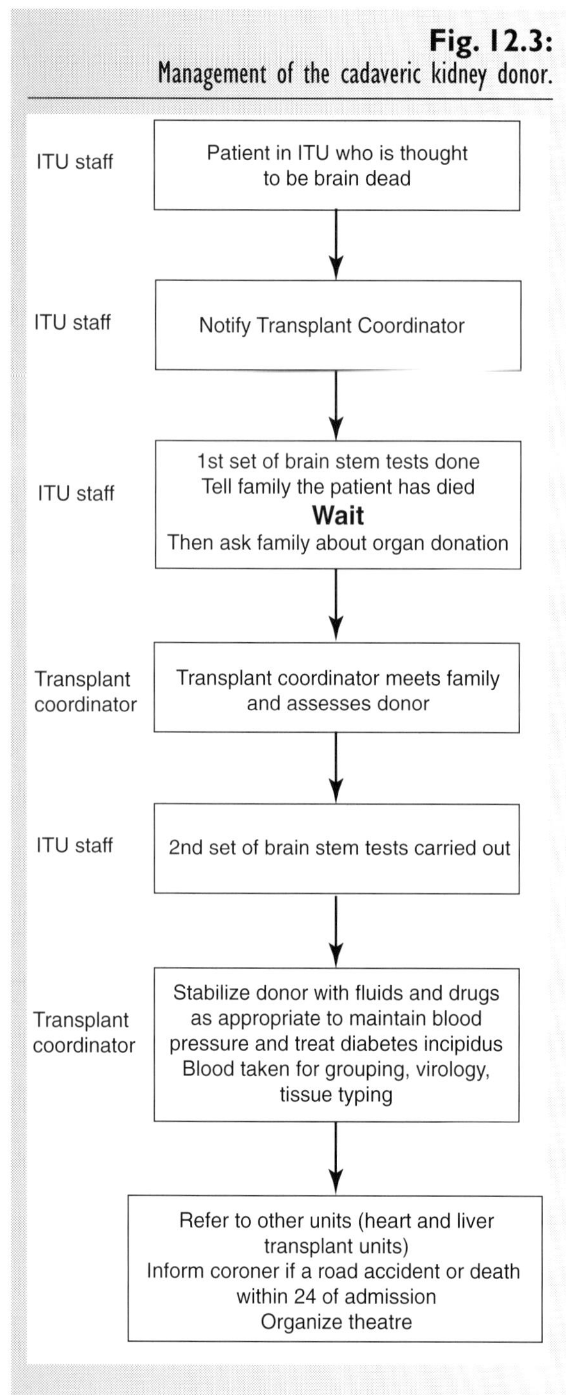

kidneys have been successfully transplanted (*Table 12.5*).

Table 12.5:
Exclusion criteria for cadaveric organ donation

1. Active sepsis
2. Viral infection e.g. HIV, hepatitis
3. Malignancy (except primary brain tumour)
4. IV drug abuse

Brain stem death

It is impossible to discuss transplantation without considering brain stem death. The majority of cadaveric donor operations are carried out on brain stem dead patients. Death can be due to intracranial or extracranial catastrophes, the latter leading to circulatory arrest which is only lethal if it lasts long enough for the brain stem to die. Thus all death is brain stem death.

It is very important to emphasize the fact that brain stem death did not evolve to satisfy the needs of transplant surgeons, but in response to the increasing medical technology that is now part and parcel of all intensive care units. If transplantation were superseded tomorrow by better treatment of organ failure, patients who are brain stem dead would still occur wherever intensive care units are established and ventilators would continue to be switched off.

The code of practice in the treatment of these patients was evolved at Harvard 1968, Minnesota 1971 and by the British Royal Colleges 1976 and 1979.

The brain stem tests are as foolproof as anything in medicine can be. They involve three phases, three 'sieves' through which the patient must pass. Firstly the diagnosis must be established, in a patient in a coma on a ventilator. Secondly endocrine, metabolic causes and the effects of drugs and hypothermia must be excluded. Only then may the tests be done. These consist of tests of apnoea and brain stem reflexes. They are done by two clinically independent doctors who have been registered for 5 years or more and have experience in intensive care. The transplant team will not be involved at this stage.

After confirming brain stem death in the cadaveric donor, a death certificate may be issued. At this stage it becomes important to manage the donor to maintain the function of the organs for transplantation. This includes monitoring and correcting physiological change associated with brain death. Thus hypotension is treated with inotropes and diabetes insipidus is treated with vasopressin.

If for any reason the organs are not going to be used, and the ventilator is turned off, one is not withdrawing treatment and allowing the patient to die, but rather stopping ventilation in someone who is already dead.

Living donor surgery

Due in part to the limited number of cadaveric organs, and in part to the increased graft survival of kidneys from living donors, the number of living related kidney transplants has increased dramatically over the last few years. The 1-year graft survival is 93% and at 5 years 85% compared with 83% and 68% respectively for first cadaveric grafts.

All operations involve some risk to life, and only in exceptional circumstances can this risk be justified in a person who is both fit and healthy. Furthermore it puts intense pressure on the surgeon who is operating on a person who does not need an operation and will not benefit physically from it.

A living related donor (LRD) donates an organ (usually a kidney) to a blood relative. This offer should come from a stable relationship, which should survive the emotional turmoil which accompanies the procedure. This may include the guilt of the recipient in putting the donor through a major operation, the feeling of superiority of the donor over the recipient. Most tragically, the guilt of the donor should the graft fail or of the recipient should the donor die from the operation (an estimated risk of 1 in 3000). Careful psychological and psychiatric assessment and counselling are crucial to allow these conflicts to be resolved satisfactorily. Living unrelated donor (LURD) transplantation is more complicated. Strictly speaking spouses fall into this category as they are not blood related, and the tissue match is unlikely to be as close as a blood relative even if the blood group is the same, but even in this situation the graft survival is better than cadaveric grafts.

Nephrectomy for a related-donor transplant can be performed via a subcostal transverse laparotomy or a loin incision. Normally the left kidney is removed, as it has a longer renal vein making the recipient operation easier. Laparoscopic donor nephrectomy is increasing in some centres, but it is important that it is carefully evaluated and is shown to be safe.

Recipient surgery

The surgical aspects of renal transplantation have not changed significantly over the last 30 years. The renal vein is anastomosed end-to-side to the external lilac vein; and the renal artery is anastomosed end to side to the external lilac artery in the case of a cadaveric organ with a Carrel (aortic) patch (*Fig. 12.4*). In the case of a living related kidney with no aortic patch, the renal artery is usually anastomosed end to end to the internal iliac artery which has been ligated distally and swung up to meet the donor renal artery. The kidney is kept cool during this period by a variety of techniques. One method is to place it in a surgical glove with the fingers tied off and surrounded by ice slush. On releasing the clamps at the end of the vascular anastomosis, the kidney is reperfused (this marks the end of the cold ischaemic time) and diuresis begins.

Fig. 12.4:
Cadaveric renal transplant.

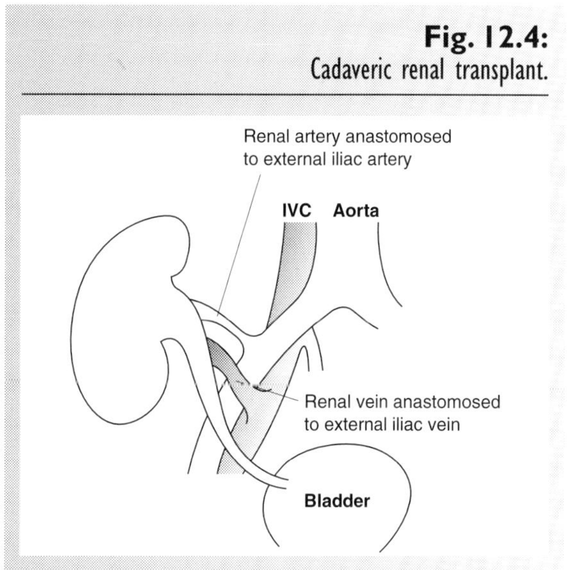

The ureter is then anastomosed to the bladder mucosa usually extravesically via an incision through the detrusor muscle and a smaller incision through the mucosa, closing the detrusor muscle over the distal ureter to prevent reflux, and protecting the anastomosis with a temporary ureteric stent.

Major urological problems seen in spina bifida, neurogenic bladder and patients with ileal conduits used to be a contra-indication to transplantation. This is no longer the case, and although graft survival may be decreased, these patients can be successfully transplanted.

Postoperative care

If the new kidney functions immediately a diuresis occurs and the appropriate fluid replacement of 50 ml plus output is initiated. A delay in the onset of function in the transplanted kidney is most frequent in those grafts experiencing a longer warm or cold ischaemia. In the early postoperative period, acute tubular necrosis (ATN) from this cause must be distinguished from other problems such as a technical error. Patients with delayed graft function have a graft biopsy to exclude rejection, an ultrasound to exclude hydronephrosis (*Fig. 12.5*) and a Doppler ultrasound to check the renal artery blood flow. They may need temporary dialysis until the kidney starts working.

Fig. 12.5: Hydronephrosis in a transplant kidney.

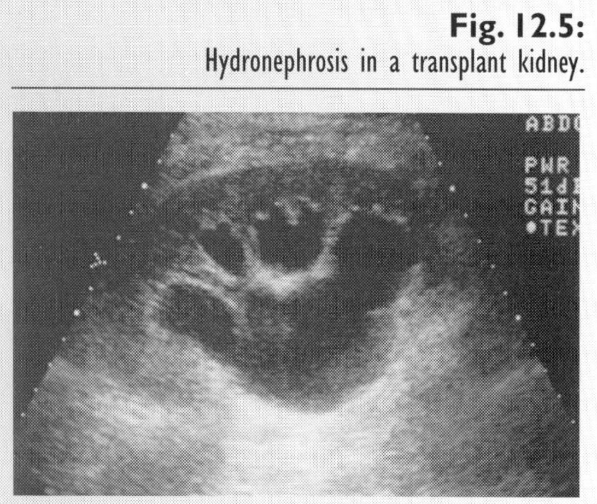

The immunology of transplantation

The most important histocompatiblity systems in renal transplantation are the **ABO blood group** and the **human leucocyte antigen** (HLA). The latter was so called because it was initially described as being present on the surface of white cells. These transplant HLA antigens are glycoproteins on the surface of cells that are coded by a group of genes known as the major histocompatibility complex (MHC) on the short arm of chromosome 6.

The MHC is polymorphic; that is to say there are multiple alleles at each locus. Over 100 HLA antigens can be detected making the HLA system the most polymorphic system found in humans. This means that in most cases it is impossible to find a fully matched donor for a particular recipient. HLA antigens are divided into two classes; class I HLA antigens are the products of the HLA-A, HLA-B and HLA-C genes, and are present on all nuclear cells of the organism. Class II HLA antigens are coded in HLA-DR, HLA-DQ and HLA-DP genes, and are mostly on the surface of B lymphocytes, activated T lymphocytes, monocytes, dendritic cells and some endothelial cells. In renal transplantation, the HLA-A, HLA-B and HLA-DR are the three most important and these antigens are routinely identified by serological methods whereby the unknown individual peripheral blood lymphocytes are incubated with antibodies directed against known alleles in the presence of complement (*Fig. 12.6*).

Binding of the specific antibody to its complementary allele causes lysis of the cells and therefore identifies the antigen. More recently, the technique of direct DNA analysis has been used. Long-term kidney survival depends on immunological compatibility between the donor and the recipient. The donor should be ABO compatible with the recipient to avoid ABO antibodies attacking graft. If there is an ABO mismatch, hyperacute or acute rejection will occur.

When matching for the MHC antigens, the class II antigens are more important than the class I antigens. Ideal matching should be identical, but this only happen between identical twins. In all other cases it should be compatible. When a donor becomes available the blood group must be compatible and then the cross-match takes place. The sites where the donor and recipient differ are

Fig. 12.6:
Serological tissue typing.

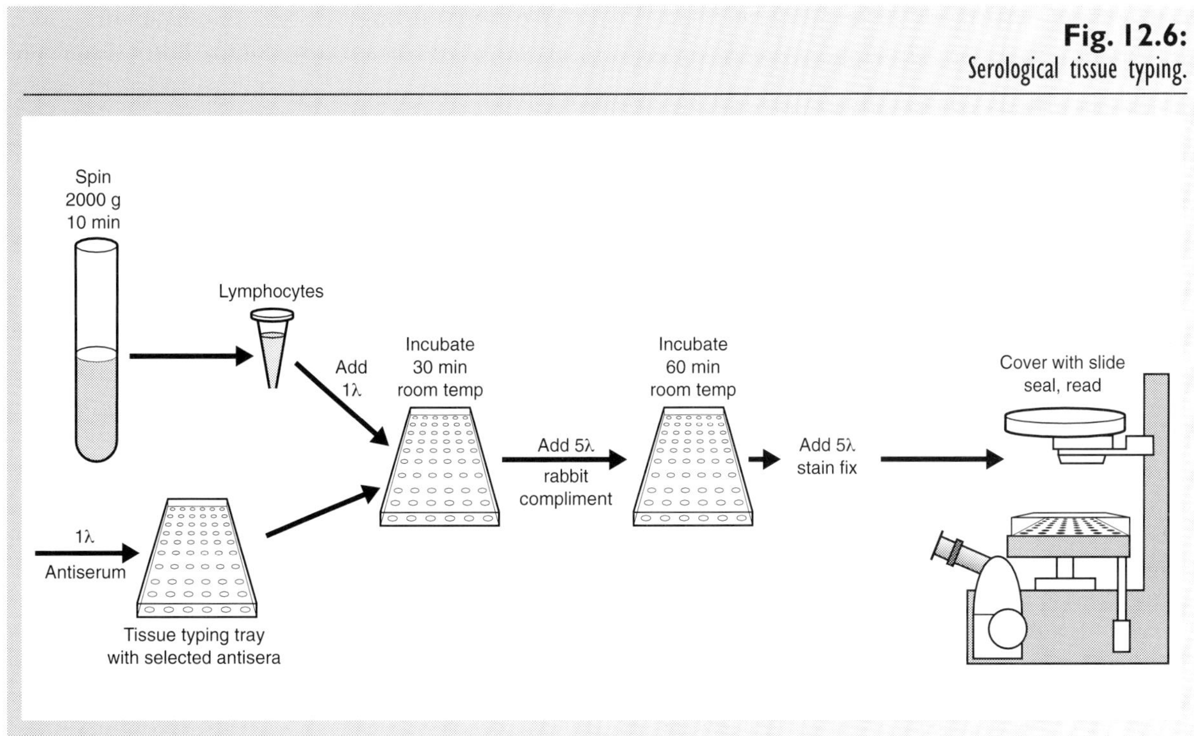

termed the mismatch and historically typing has reported on the mismatches rather than the matches. In the example in *Table 12.6a* this would be reported as a 1-1-1 mismatch, while *Table 12.6b* would be reported as a 1-0-0 mismatch

Cross-matching should give a negative result. The recipient serum and the donor's lymphocytes (spleen cells or lymph node cells) are used in setting up the crossmatch. Recipient antibodies will bind to donor and lyse the donor cells if the crossmatch is positive or this can also now be detected by flow cytometry.

Sensitization of the recipient is of great importance for the outcome of the transplant. If there are cytotoxic antibodies in the recipient's serum due to exposure to HLA antigens in blood transfusions, pregnancy or previous transplants this may lead to anti-HLA antibodies and a patient who will be sensitized. The degree of sensitization allows a prediction of the probability of a positive outcome of the cross-match test between the donor and recipient.

Table 12.6a:
Example of a 1-1-1 mismatch

	A	B	DR
Donor	1,4	3,7	3,4
Recipient	1,3	3,8	4,6
Mismatch	1	1	1

Table 12.6b:
Example of a 1-0-0 mismatch

	A	B	DR
Donor	1,4	3,8	2,3
Recipient	1,3	3,8	2,3
Mismatch	1	0	0

Rejection

Hyperacute rejection occurs within minutes of transplanting and occurs due to pre-formed HLA antibodies or as a result of ABO blood group incompatibility. Preformed antibodies bind to graft endothelial cells of vessels resulting in complement activation and sludging and thrombosis within vessels. Histologically microthrombi and polymorphs are in abundance.

Acute rejection may be vascular or cell mediated and usually occurs within days or weeks but may occur at any time post-transplant (for example if the patient stops taking immunosuppressive therapy. There is a marked lymphocytic infiltration in the tubules and vessels of the transplanted kidney, which cause subsequent damage.

Classification of acute cellular rejection is carried out according to the Banff criteria, which is based on the degree of lymphocytic infiltration of the tubules, endothelial cells and vasculature.

Chronic rejection may occur months or years post-transplant and is characterized by progressive intimal proliferation, interstitial fibrosis with a gradual deterioration in graft function.

Immunosuppression

Apart from the notable exception of transplants between identical twins, continued immunosuppression is inevitable for the long-term function of transplanted organs. An acute rejection episode is a feature of 40–45% of renal transplant patients, and is detrimental to the function and outcome of renal allografts. The objective of immunosuppression is to prevent graft rejection while maintaining the immunological function of the recipient to its maximum effect.

Immunosuppressive protocols differ between centres, but the drugs are the same. The different groups and their actions are outlined in *Table 12.7*.

The basic immunosuppressive drugs after transplantation are corticosteroids, azathioprine, cyclosporine. Triple therapy using these three or their newer alternatives is standard immunosuppressive practice in many centres (*Table 12.8*).

Corticosteroids have been part of the immunosuppressive treatment after renal transplants from the beginning, as well as being used during rejection episodes. Their mechanism of action is the inhibition of T lymphocyte activation by blocking the expression of the IL-1 and IL-6 genes. Because of their known side effects, lower doses are now used which has dramatically reduced the incidence of postoperative complications. Azathioprine is a derivative of 6-mercaptopurine; it inhibits the synthesis of purines and the formation of RNA, blocking the proliferation of T lymphocytes. The most significant side effects of azathioprine are the depression of bone marrow and hepatotoxicity.

Cyclosporine was introduced into clinical practice in 1976; it is a cyclic polypeptide of fungal origin and was an important step towards improving the results of organ transplantation. Cyclosporine inhibits IL-2-dependent proliferation of activated T-cells. It is nephrotoxic to the kidney and its blood

Table 12.7:
Four groups of immunosuppressive drugs

Drug	Action
Steroid	Blocks inflammatory response (IL-1, IL-6 gene expression)
Cyclosporine, tacrolimus, rapamycin	Blocks IL-2 production
Azathioprine, mycophenolate	Anti-proliferative (inhibits purine synthesis)
Polyclonal antibody (anti thymocyte globulin)	Anti-T cell
Monoclonal antibody OKT3	

Table 12.8:
Immunosuppression regimens for use in the standard situation and acute rejection

Clinical situation	Immunosuppression
Standard immunosuppression 'triple therapy'	Cyclosporine (or tacrolimus or rapamycin) Azathioprine (or mycophenolate) Corticosteroids
Acute rejection	(a) Methylprednisolone (b) Polyclonal antibody (c) Monoclonal antibody (d) Tacrolimus 'rescue'

levels need monitoring. Cyclosporine toxicity is one cause of impaired renal function post-transplantation, and has been the cause of renal failure in patients who have had other organ transplants.

In the 1960s, a polyclonal antibody, antithymocyte globulin (ATG) was developed for use from sera derived from horses or rabbits immunized with human lymphoid tissue for use both in prevention and for the treatment of steroid-resistant rejection. The immunosuppressive effect of polyclonal immunoglobulins lies in the depletion of T lymphocytes. Because the effects of particular polyclonal antibodies are not consistent, mouse-derived monoclonal antibodies directed against the CD3 antigen complex on all mature human T cells were developed at the end of the 1970s. As they have several serious side effects, their main use is in the treatment of steroid-resistant rejection.

Tacrolimus and rapamycin are macrolide antibiotics with a similar action and side effects to cyclosporine but much more potent. Their main advantage after renal transplantation is in the ability to reduce the dose of corticosteroids.

Mycophenolate is an anti-metabolite with a similar action to azathioprine and is now being increasingly used as an alternative to azathioprine, particularly after the first rejection episode.

Complications of transplantation

Complications of transplantation may be due to surgical or immunological aspects.

Patients undergoing renal transplantation often have multiple medical problems associated with dialysis, renal failure uraemia and immunosuppression. After cardiovascular causes, infections are the next most frequent cause of mortality following transplantation. In the early days of transplantation when high-dose steroids were common practice, these complications were much higher.

The incidence of **urological** complications after renal transplantation varies but is usually between 5–10%. The two most common urological complications are obstruction and fistula formation from the lower end of the ureter. These develop because of damage to the ureteric blood supply during organ removal. In the normal anatomical situation, the blood supply of the ureter comes from the renal artery, the iliac vessels and the superior vesical artery. After removal it is entirely dependent on the renal artery, and this is why it is essential to remove the ureter with a good supply of adventitia surrounding it. Obstruction and fistula can be dealt with by a variety of endoscopic procedures using ureteric stents inserted in an antegrade or retrograde fashion (*Fig. 12.7*). If this is not successful open surgery may be needed to reimplant the ureter, or use the native ureter to by-pass the obstruction. With proper urological management, the chance of saving the graft is very high. Vesico-ureteric reflux is common after transplantation (*Fig. 12.8*). This is not important if the urine is sterile. Lymphoceles may sometimes cause ureteral obstruction. Most cases occur within 6 months of transplantation. The classic triad at presentation is decreased urine output, hydronephrosis and ipsilateral leg oedema. Treatment in the first instance

Fig. 12.7:
Antegrade pyelogram showing ureteric obstruction in a transplant kidney which has a nephrostomy tube in situ. A CAPD catheter is still in position.

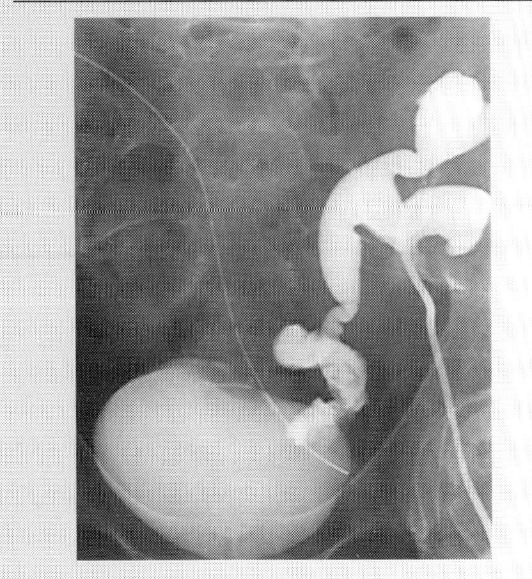

Fig. 12.8:
Micturating cystogram showing vesico-ureteric reflux in both native kidneys and the transplant kidney

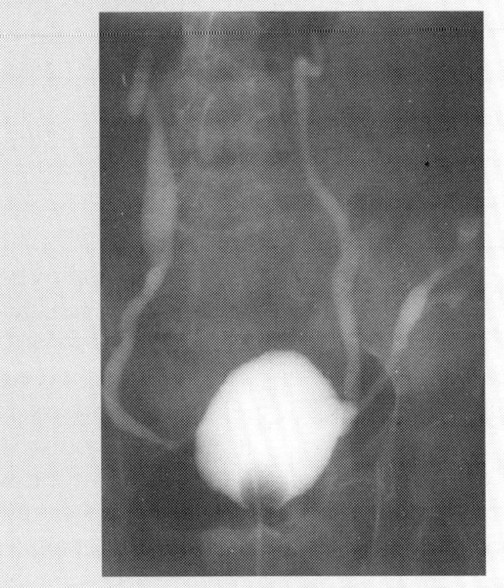

involves aspiration, but if recurring, fenestration into the peritoneal cavity is performed at open operation or by endoscopic techniques

Vascular complications include bleeding, renal vein thrombosis which although rare can lead to graft rupture; renal artery stenosis can be corrected by transluminal angioplasty.

The most significant **nonsurgical** complications after renal transplantation are infections and malignancies. Both are due to the effects of immunosuppression. Infections can be bacterial, viral, fungal or protozoal. Viral infections can be caused by cytomegalovirus (CMV), Epstein-Barr virus and hepatitis viruses. Kidneys from hepatitis-positive donors should not be used. CMV alone causes symptomatic diseases in 35% and death in 2% of patients after renal transplantation. If a kidney from a CMV-positive donor is transplanted, an antiviral agent such as gancyclovir is administered to the recipient.

Malignancy is a complication of the immunosuppressed state of the recipient, the common ones being skin cancers and lymphoma.

Results of transplantation

Figure 12.9 shows the renal graft survival of over 1000 patients treated at the Oxford transplant centre since 1985 who were given triple therapy (cyclosporine, azathioprine and prednisolone) for

Fig. 12.9:
Renal graft survival with triple therapy (1985–1999) in the Oxford Transplant Centre.

--- First grafts (997)
— Second grafts (167)
Percent survival
100
80
60
40
20
0
0 1 2 3 4 5 6 7 8 9 10
Years

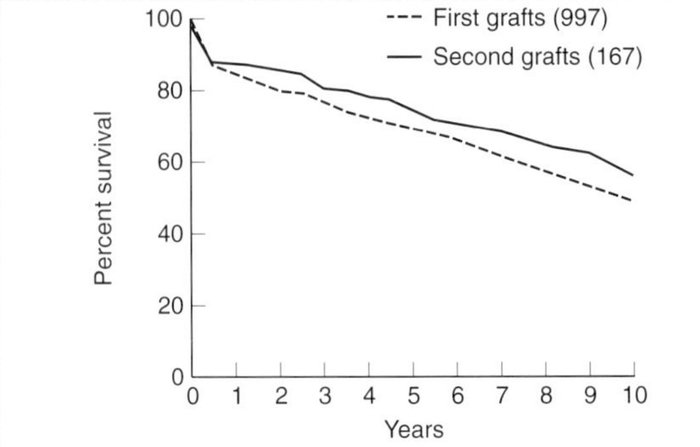

immunosuppression. The 1-year graft survival for first grafts is 85% and at 5 years this drops to 75% for first graft and 70% for second grafts. The graft survival for living-related donors is higher with over 90% 1-year survival and over 80% 5-year survival. With newer forms of immunosuppression the figures should continue to improve. The initial sharp drop from 100% in the first 6 months is due to the complications of the transplant operation itself and early rejection.

Key points

- Sudden anuria is likely to represent a post-renal obstruction to the outflow of urine rather than a renal cause.
- The most important histocompatibility systems in renal transplantation are the ABO blood group and the human leucocyte antigen (HLA).
- The genes that code for the HLA antigens are known as the major histocompatibility complex (MHC) and are found on the short arm of chromosome 6.
- Blood transfusions, pregnancy or previous transplants may lead to anti-HLA antibodies and a patient who will be sensitized.
- A standard immunosuppression regimen after transplantation is triple therapy with cyclosporine, azathioprine and prednisolone.
- Major congenital urological abnormalities are no longer a contra-indication to transplantation.
- Complications of transplant surgery are best prevented by meticulous attention to detail than cured later.
- After transplantation the blood supply to the ureter is entirely dependent on the renal artery.
- The common urological complications are obstruction and fistula due to ischaemia of the lower ureter.
- The common non-surgical complications of transplantation are infection and malignancy due to immunosuppression.
- Kidney transplants from living donors have a better outcome than from cadaveric donors.

Cases

1. A 29-year-old motor cyclist has been admitted to the intensive care unit following a major road traffic accident. He remains in a coma after neuro-surgical exploration and his outlook is bleak. He carries an organ donor card.
   (a) Which steps need to be taken before organ donation is carried out?
   (b) With whom can the neurosurgical SHO carry out the brain death tests?
   (c) What needs to be said to the family?
   (d) Which contra-indications might there be to organ donation?

2. A 50-year-old woman had her first renal transplant 2 weeks ago. Her creatinine initially came down from 850 mmol l^{-1} to 150 and now it has risen to 230.
   (a) What are the possible causes?
   (b) Which investigations would you arrange?
   (c) What is the first line of treatment for acute rejection?
   (d) What are the complications of transplant biopsy?

3. A 60-year-old man wishes to donate a kidney to his wife.
   (a) Is this allowed?
   (b) What preoperative investigations does he need?
   (c) Is his life expectancy altered after donating a kidney?
   (d) What are the chance of it being successful?

Answers

1. (a) Firstly the diagnosis of brain death must be established. The brain stem tests are not carried out unless the patient is in a coma on a ventilator and endocrine, metabolic causes and the effects of drugs and hypothermia have been excluded. Brain stem testing is carried out whether or not organ donation is going to proceed. The situation needs full discussion with the family. The transplant

unit and in particular the transplant co-ordinator is contacted.

(b) A neurosurgical SHO cannot carry out brain death tests unless he or she has been registered for 5 years or more. Guidelines advise that the diagnosis should be made by two independent doctors, one a consultant experienced in intensive care or acute medicine.

(c) Although the patient carried an organ donor card, the family should still be asked about organ donation, and while they will not usually object it is not the policy to over-rule the wishes of the relatives.

(d) Active sepsis, HIV or hepatitis infections, any malignancy except primary brain tumour and low grade skin tumours, intravenous drug abuse.

2. (a) The common causes are acute rejection, ureteric obstruction and cyclosporine toxicity.

(b) Investigations should include ultrasound of the kidney, and renal biopsy and cyclosporine blood levels.

(c) The first line of treatment for acute rejection is pulsed intravenous methyl prednisolone.

(d) Transplant biopsy is not without its complications and can cause haematuria and a subcapsular or perinephric haematoma. In 1 in 4000 cases it can lead to graft loss.

3. (a) Yes. Living unrelated kidney donation is allowed, but in the UK there is a regulatory body that looks at every case of unrelated donation and gives or refuses permission.

(b) He will need a full medical examination with particular attention being paid to past medical history, renal and cardiac function. Routine blood screening tests. Creatinine clearance, chest X-ray, assessment of the arterial supply, venous and ureteric drainage of the kidneys. An assessment of his emotional and psychiatric state is important. He must be made aware of the risk of surgical complications and a very small (1 in 3000) risk of death. He must also be made aware that there is a small chance the kidney will not function and in the case of serious complications may need to be removed.

(c) His actuarial life expectance is actually improved after kidney donation. This is because he has successfully completed extensive medical screening tests before being allowed to donate a kidney, and major medical problems have been excluded at this stage. There is no evidence of any detrimental long-term effect to the donor as a result of giving a kidney.

(d) Living unrelated transplants are more successful than cadaveric transplants. The 1-year graft survival is 90% and the 5-year graft survival is 80%.

Further Reading

Morris P.J. (2000) *Kidney Transplantation, Principles and Practice.* Fifth edition. W.B. Saunders, Philadelphia.

Resnick M.D. and Novick A.C. (1995) *Urology Secrets.* Hanley & Belfus, Philadelphia.

Morris P.J. (2000) *UK living related donor guidelines.* Report of the British Transplantation Society, London.

Index